Simple Advice

By James O. Page

Simple Advice

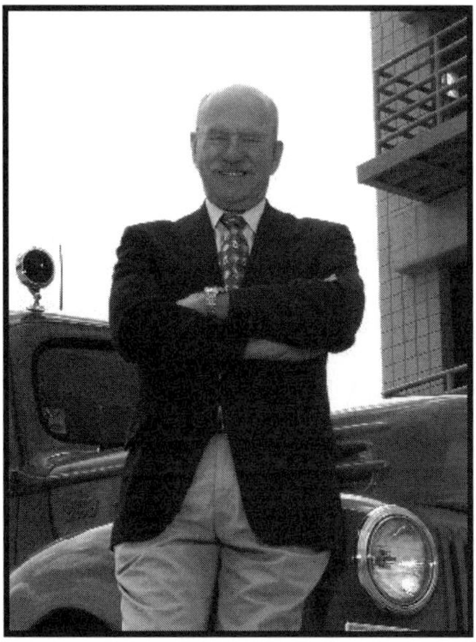

Publisher Emeritus/Founder
Jems Communications/FireRescue
Magazine.

Published by:
Jems Communications, FireRescue Magazine

Publisher:
Jeff Berend

Book Design:
Jason Pelc

Cover Design:
Janene Long-Forman, John Fattahi

Production:
Janene Long-Forman

ISBN: 0-936174-14-5

FireRescue Magazine is published by:
Jems Communications
1947 Camino Vida Roble. Ste. 200
Carlsbad, CA 92008
760/431-9797 FAX 760/431-8176
www.jems.com

Printed and bound in the United States of America.

Cover: Jim Page and grandson Kenny in front of Rescue 11. Photo by Tom Page.

More than 4,800 American firefighters have died in the line of duty since I first earned the right to call myself a firefighter. The public respect and adoration that we now enjoy was paid for with those priceless lives. With humility and appreciation, we dedicate this book to the memory of those who made the ultimate sacrifice.

James O. Page

November 2001

Contents

Foreword

As a junior-level editor, I wasn't allowed to touch Jim Page's columns. The more senior editors assured me I didn't yet have the editing chops. A few years later, I was finally deemed ready.

I sat down with my pencil sharpened, ready to go to work. As I read line after line, the realization hit me: editing Jim Page's writing is an incredibly difficult task. Difficult because there's nothing to edit (those senior editors were pretty smart!).

That's because his words are woven as tightly as Egyptian cotton. Every sentence and phrase is placed so perfectly that to change it would be an unthinkable act. That can make an editor feel a little redundant—but it sure makes for a great read.

My guess is that his writing style is both natural and intentional. Jim likely learned early on when writing for fire service magazines—not to mention city managers and councils—that the best way to guarantee no one messes with your stuff is to make it perfect from the start.

Even more important than style is the story. And Jim Page tells damn good stories. He's got literally thousands of them, each with amazing twists and profound lessons. Those stories are equally riveting in writing as they are spoken, and that's pretty unusual. There are a lot of great speakers who can't write, and great writers who can't speak—Jim does both with an ability that leaves his readers and listeners both humbled and inspired.

I'm sure Jim's experience as an attorney plays a significant role in his storytelling and oratory ability. (He finished law school and became a member of the California Bar in 1971 while working for the L.A. County Fire Department.) There's nothing that can make a judge or jury glaze over more quickly than technical-speak with no personal connection. But a story about a person with a face and a name pulls you in and makes you listen (and read).

It's no different for members of the fire service. Take the firefighter recruit, overwhelmed by fire flow formulas, street maps and volumes of information. Textbooks and training are important, but at the forefront of that recruit's mind will be the stories his company officer told him and their vital lessons.

Over the course of more than 40 years in the fire service, including tenures as a chief in three departments, Jim has become—in the opinions of many based on the letters we get—one of the fire service's most prolific storytellers. Why are his stories so entertaining and educational? He's a tremendous listener (a good lesson to all of us), and has an almost machine-like ability to remember facts, figures, dates and people. Walk around a major fire conference with Jim and you'll realize it's not an exaggeration to say Jim knows literally thousands of regular fire folks and legends alike by name (and at least one story about each of them).

These stories offer important lessons for all of us. It really is simple advice, but it's the most important advice one can receive. And from James O. Page, one of the 20th century's most influential fire service luminaries, it really means something.

I've had the pleasure and honor of being the first person to read many of these stories as they came off Jim's office printer. I gratefully accepted the fact that there isn't any editing to do on his essays a long time ago. I suggest you do what I do: sit back and enjoy the read.

Jeff Berend
November 2001

Preface

Fires and rescues are a writer's cornucopia. They are events filled with danger, bravery, conflict, action, intrigue, excitement, frustration, and sometimes even humor. The people who fight fires and perform rescues are tall and short, lean and fat, young and old, handsome and homely, and every degree of variation between the extremes. Day in and day out, they go to places others run from, and they do things others could never dream of doing.

For my entire adult life, it's been my good fortune to live and work in America's diverse community of firefighters and rescuers. They accepted me as a young recruit, and they tolerated me as I learned the tricks of their trade and the intricacies of their culture. They taught me the arts and sciences of fire and rescue, and they ultimately promoted me to positions of leadership. In the process I absorbed the culture and values of these courageous helpers and care-givers.

More than 30 years ago, I first published some impressions and opinions about emergency services and the people of fire and rescue. That was more than 350 published articles and columns ago. In those articles and columns I've praised people and events when warranted. I've scolded on occasion. I've tried to shed light on organizational behavior, faulty leadership, bureaucratic nonsense and irresponsible journalists. I've shared a lot of personal stories from throughout my career.

It started with a column in The Nozzle, the newsletter of

firefighters' union Local 1014, and occasional articles in the monthly magazine, Straight Streams, published by and for Los Angeles County firefighters. In the 1970s I wrote regular columns in several EMS newsletter publications and in a new magazine devoted to paramedics. In 1979 we founded JEMS (Journal of Emergency Medical Services) and started buying ink by the barrel. In 1988 we created Rescue Magazine, which we later merged with another publication to form FireRescue Magazine.

Soon after launching JEMS, we learned that our readers rated my monthly column as a "must read" feature. Since then, I've traveled far and wide with open eyes and ears, searching for relevant, interesting topics and issues to share with readers. I've never taken my readers for granted, and I humbly appreciate their interest in my writing, even when they disagree.

In 1986, we packaged 39 of my columns and essays into a book that was named "The Magic of 3AM." It was very popular for a dozen years and through five printings.

The editors of FireRescue Magazine suggested we create another book of selected columns. The 45 essays contained in this book, "Simple Advice," were chosen. Each of them represents my efforts to inform, educate and entertain with a simple formula - plain truth and common sense. I hope you enjoy the book.

James O. Page
November 2001

1

One Man's Career

My Greatest Legal Victory

Every lawyer keeps a mental tally of his or her worst defeats and greatest victories. Most of the defeats are delivered by a judge or jury. Most of the victories have something to do with money. Not mine.

The lady arrived without an appointment. I recognized her name and told the receptionist I'd meet with her. As she walked into my office, she was tense and unsmiling. After she was seated, I inquired about her name.

"Are you married to..."

"Yes," she interrupted. "I know you used to work together, and I don't know any other lawyers. I'm sorry I didn't call first."

Without fanfare, she told me that she wanted to file for divorce. "I'm tired of being a 'widow'," she said. "When he's not on duty, he's volunteering as a course instructor. When he's home, he's always on the phone lining up new courses to teach or solving other people's problems. Or he's out in the garage working on his equipment or inventing some new rescue device. There's never any time for me and the kids."

I then asked one of those questions you have to ask in the divorce business: "Is there another man in your life?"

"No!" she exclaimed, and broke into tears.

"To your knowledge, is there another woman in his life," I asked. "I almost wish there was," she said, dabbing at her wet eyes. "I wouldn't like it, but I could almost understand it if he was having an affair with a woman. I could compete with another woman, but I can't compete with all of this fire and rescue stuff."

She continued to share with me the frustrations that had driven her to consider divorce. Her husband was highly respected by his colleagues. He was well known throughout the area for his knowledge and skills, his ability to teach others, and his boundless dedication. Like many of us, however, he hadn't convinced his family that he was also dedicated to them.

A few days earlier, I had completed a continuing legal education (CLE) course on family law. It included some valuable information from a marriage and family counselor. I learned that we all have some very basic psychological needs, such as identity, stimulation, security and a sense of self-worth.

A few more questions revealed that the young wife and mother loved her man very much. She didn't really want a divorce, I concluded. Probably, she was trying to use me to get a message to him. Instead of explaining the divorce process, I shared with her some of the lessons I'd learned in the CLE course, and applied those lessons to her husband's other passion.

He had achieved one of his basic needs-identity-by being the best in his field. Mention his name among colleagues and everybody knew who you were talking about. What's more, everybody mentioned his name with the respect that's shown for a special few.

Another of the needs-stimulation-is an individual thing. I suppose there are accountants who get stimulated by income tax returns and lawyers who get stimulated by drafting wills and trusts. But this lady and her children shared the life of a guy whose need for stimulation required much greater personal challenge. As we talked about it, she agreed that was one of the things she found most attractive about him. Her man was not dull or boring. Of course, he was not around much, either.

The third need-security-was met when he found his useful place in society, and when others appreciated him for what he could do. As long as a fire station or a rescue squad was nearby, he would never be far from friends. Somehow, he hadn't recognized the security that waited for him at home.

The sense of self-worth, the fourth of our basic needs, was probably the driving force that propelled the man to work so hard in service to others. The problem was, he seldom included his family among the "others." A bigger problem was that his wife had lost her sense of self-worth.

While the woman was in my office, I called the counselor who had taught the family law course. It became a conference call and we all agreed that divorce was premature. We made an appointment for the couple to visit the counselor, but it was the wife's job to get her husband there.

It worked. The man took on his biggest rescue-saving his marriage. He began to share more of his life with his family, and he learned to help his wife meet her basic psychological needs, especially the sense of self-worth. But she also learned to appreciate his world, and she found ways to be part of it.

There was another word that the counselor mentioned: "balance." Above all, we need balance in our lives. I was able to steer a rescuer and his family toward the help they needed to bring balance into their lives. And I consider that to be my greatest victory as a lawyer.

Kerosene Rags

I thought when you joined the fire department that you'd come home smelling like smoke," my wife announced as she loaded the Maytag. "Instead, your work clothes reek of kerosene." I explained to her that we used kerosene on wiping rags when we went under the rigs every afternoon. "You wipe down the underside of your fire trucks?" she asked incredulously. "Sure," I replied. "It's a fire service tradition. We try to make 'em shine on the bottom just like they do on top."

"That's ridiculous," she declared. "Nobody's gonna look under a truck to see if it's shiny. Why don't you just steam clean all the greasy stuff underneath every 90 days or so?" "I'll ask the chief...uh, after I get about 10 years of seniority," I replied.

She planted the seeds of dissent. For several months, as I rolled the creeper around under Engine 2, with a portable light in one hand and a kerosene-soaked rag in the other, I mumbled, "This is a ridiculous waste of time and talent."

Then one day, while I was reaching up into the unseen nooks and crannies of a rear spring mount bracket, the rag caught on something sharp. I ran my bare index finger over the same area and felt a thin, ragged edge that ran from one side of the cast iron bracket to the other. There was no way to get a good look at it but I suspected that the bracket had fractured.

The Captain checked for himself and confirmed my suspicion. The rig was taken out of service immediately. The broken spring hanger was replaced within a few days. I received an "Attaboy" from the chief. A potentially horrible accident was avoided, and I was able to tell my wife why that old fire service tradition also made sense.

That was a long time ago. Now, fire apparatus is better built, safer, sturdier, more durable, and easier to drive. The fire rigs of today go faster and stop quicker, they cost a lot more and-with the almost universal adoption of medical first response-they're a lot busier.

In visiting fire stations around the country, I've noticed that some departments take their modern fire apparatus pretty much for granted.

"How do you like the Cummins?" I asked one engine driver as we surveyed his year-old quarter-million-dollar quint.

"What do you mean?" he asked.

"The power plant that motates this thing."

"I never noticed what it was," he explained. "I just step on the gas and it goes."

Coincidentally, the lug nuts on his wheels were caked with scuzz, the inboard corners of the diamond-plate steps were filled with old dirt and road grime, and there were some empty soda cans rolling around on the floor of the cab.

Hand tools and salvage equipment had remnants of soot and mud from long-forgotten fires.

I don't mean to sound like some old fart with a fetish for kerosene, but what's the deal with filthy, unkempt fire apparatus? How can firefighters be proud of themselves if the horse they ride's been used hard and put away dirty?

Let's start with the basics. The fire department is the community's last resort for some of the worst kinds of bad things that happen. Like big fires and train wrecks and building collapses-the kinds of things the cops are running away from when you arrive. Who else can they call if the fire department can't handle it?

In most communities the local fire company is the basic resource for fire protection, emergency medical services, and disaster response. The local fire company depends on a mobile platform (pumper or ladder apparatus) to get to where it can do its job with the needed people, tools and equipment. In other words, a fire company is nothing without safe and reliable wheels.

Some of our ancestors were pretty smart, actually. When the old-timers sent us under the rigs with kerosene rags, they knew that frequent inspection of mechanical equipment inevitably will reveal problems that can be fixed before they cause further harm. Many of them grew up on farms, and they knew that clean equipment will last longer and be more reliable than dirty equipment. Most of them had rebuilt an automobile engine or two, and packed a few wheel bearings. They knew that friction is the enemy of all mechanical equipment. Dirt between moving surfaces magnifies the damage.

The reliability of mechanical equipment is directly related to the quality and frequency of maintenance. The best example is United Parcel Service. Some of those shiny brown trucks are more than 30 years old, and you seldom see one being towed home. UPS has one of the world's best preventive maintenance programs, just so they can get our packages to us on time.

A real pro treats tools of the trade with pride and tender loving care, especially when lives depend on it. When you step into a scruffy, dirty elevator, do you wonder about the machinery you can't see? If you had your choice of taxicabs to ride in, would you pick a dirty one or a clean one? When you board an airliner, do you expect the pilot to know a lot about the engines? What if he said, "I just open the throttles and it goes."

We've heard a lot about the need to change, and to abandon many of our fire service traditions. Well, there are a few traditions that we need to preserve-or, in some cases, get back to.

I Saved That Building

About five years into my career, I gave up a coveted spot at a busy fire station to volunteer for a 40-hour-a-week job as a fire prevention inspector. The guys at 29's were convinced I was crazy. Wear a white shirt and a tie every day? Shuffle paper and write reports? Give up all the fun and games at the station to work for Francis McCarthy? "He's nuts!" they concluded.

I was looking for an opportunity to learn. Capt. McCarthy was in charge of a fire prevention district that included every known fire hazard, from rundown housing and illicit auto repair shops to an auto assembly plant, several chemical manufacturers and hundreds of businesses run by immigrant merchants. The training started on my first day. "Mac," as we called him, handed me an inspection report and a clipboard. As we covered every inch of a metal fabrication factory, he reeled off code violations: "Southwest corner of mezzanine, north machine shop area, provide approved electrical outlet per section 26485 of fire code. Eliminate extension cord wiring."

The inspection took two full days. Mac could spot violations from 200' and he knew the code sections from memory. The inspection report ran 36 pages long. My thumb and index finger were grooved from pressing through the carbon copies. My head was full of new information. I missed the fire station, to be sure, but every day for the next two years would be a learning experience.

Capt. McCarthy was an old bachelor who'd saved three cents of every nickel he ever earned. Aside from salty language and bad jokes in inappropriate situations, his worst characteristic was the cheap cigars he smoked. The headliner and the windows of his staff sedan (a hand-me-down from a Battalion Chief) had a greenish-brown cast from the constant cloud of cigar smoke. But he knew the fire code and the building code and the electrical code, and he didn't mind teaching what he knew to a "young smart-ass" (which is what he called me).

About a year into my internship with Capt. McCarthy, I realized that he detested re-inspections, so he never did them. He enjoyed the hunt for violations. He liked to compile great lists of those violations, especially if he could get a new inspector to do the writing. More than anything, he seemed to enjoy delivering his inspection notices to plant managers, business owners, shop superintendents, etc. But then he never went back to see whether they had complied.

My time with Francis McCarthy paid off when I took the next three promotional exams. I had learned more than I realized. The day-to-day exposure to all the stuff of fire prevention prepared me for exam questions that left others scratching their heads. To this day, I cannot walk through a factory building without looking for fire code violations.

Still, in most fire departments, prevention doesn't get the respect it deserves. Usually, there are people who have the responsibility for such things as plan checks, business licenses and annual occupancy inspections, and special permit and licensing activities. Some people really like doing those things and have built their careers around fire prevention. Others are assigned to "the bureau" for varying periods of time; usually, they have a calendar on their desk with the remaining days of their assignment numbered. Out in the stations, however, fire prevention doesn't generate a whole lot of excitement.

It's kinda like the difference between a State Department diplomat and a Special Forces commando. One is prepared to prevent war, and the other's ready to wage it. Another example is the difference between a public health physician and a trauma surgeon. In the police business, an example is the difference between a crime prevention team and a SWAT team.

One day while inspecting an old movie theater, I found a cheap, frayed extension cord running beneath a section of the heavy, velvet stage curtain. The building was unsprinklered, and most of the fire extinguishers had been stolen. The flame-proofing tag on the curtain indicated that it had not been treated for several years beyond the deadline. "Fire Prevention Inspector Saves Lives of Dozens," the headline could have read. But, of course, it didn't. Prevention doesn't make headlines.

Another day, while inspecting a metal plating plant, I discovered a poisonous solution in a glass coffeepot on a hot plate-directly adjacent to a pot of real coffee. It had never occurred to the shop foreman that somebody might fill their cup from the wrong pot. That night, as I watched the TV news, I indulged myself in a fantasy: "NBC presents: 'Death Defied, the True Story of a Diligent Fire Prevention Inspector and How He Saved an Unsuspecting Factory Worker from the Grim Reaper.'" Of course, that would never happen. Prevention is not the stuff of fantasies.

Capt. McCarthy usually sent one of his inspectors into attics, cellars or other places one was likely to find spiders or rodents. One day, he dispatched me to inspect the attic of a wing of classrooms in a 50-year-old high school. I found plenty of spiders, and some dead rats, but I also found an overheated electrical wire stapled to a wooden rafter. The wood was already slightly charred. We demanded that it be fixed before we left the building. Even now, every time I drive by the school, I think, "I saved that building," or "I cheated Engine 3 out of a humongous fire."

At the end of my two years in the fire prevention bureau, I could look on the experience with pride. I knew I had saved more lives and preserved more property than if I had spent 10 years on a busy engine company. But, instead of headlines and valor awards, the evidence was all on paper, stored in filing cabinets for nobody to see. Furthermore, the guys at 29's still thought I was crazy for volunteering to work in fire prevention.

We know that preventing fires-and the deaths, injuries and property losses-is our first and most important responsibility. But it's hard work, and it's getting more and more complicated all the time.. There's another side of this business that needs attention and respect. Next time you see your fire marshal (or some firefighter who's volunteered to spend a year or two in the fire prevention bureau) let them know that what they do is important.

The Grandest Parade

One long-standing tradition in Southern California has always made me a little uncomfortable: the Tournament of Roses Parade and the Rose Bowl Game. Why? These events always take place on New Year's Day when the weather in SoCal is almost always perfect.

I might better describe my discomfort as empathy. The genetic influence of my Scottish Presbyterian ancestors compels me to care about those less fortunate. Thus, when I see and hear weather reports from the frigid two-thirds of the continent, I empathize with those who watch the warm, sunny parade and football game on TV while their own weather outside is unbearable.

I've actually been in the Tournament of Roses Parade twice. The first time, at age 14, I was third trumpet in the Los Angeles County Sheriff's Boys Band. On Jan. 1, 2001, I was one of seven guys in period costume pushing and pulling an antique hand pumper (circa 1853) along the 4.6-mile parade route. On both occasions, the air was clear and dry, and the temperature was in the mid-70s.

If you saw this year's parade on NBC, you missed us. The director cut to Al Roker for a weather report and commercial break just as we pushed our 1,500-pound rig past the cameras. That's OK-several hundred thousand people cheered us on. Their generous appreciation helped me to forget all about my gimpy knee.

I participated in this year's parade with the County of Los Angeles Fire Museum Association. The California State Firefighters Association (CSFA) Steamer Team invited us to join as part of a five-unit display of fire service history. In addition to our hand pumper, a hand-drawn hose cart and three horse-drawn rigs took part-the CSFA steamer, a San Bernardino hose wagon and a Fresno ladder truck. The matched black Percherons and the white Shire draft horses were a show all by themselves, but they sure left a mess in the street.

In show business, they say you should never appear with dogs or kids because they'll always upstage you. Dave Hubert, owner and operator of the CSFA steamer, walked the parade with his well-trained dalmatian Blaze. She charmed the crowds and the TV cameras-mooching a few snacks along the way.

Every entry in the Rose Parade must be decorated with flowers. The night before the parade, we received buckets of leftover flowers from float builders. A bunch of hairy-chested firefighters got busy demonstrating previously unknown talents as they fashioned wreaths and garlands for our old rigs. Finally, we hung four buckets of red-and-white, long-stemmed carnations and roses from the handrails. Along the parade route, we took turns jogging to the edge of the crowd to hand the long-stem flowers to pretty little girls or little old ladies in wheelchairs. The crowds roared with approval.

The half-mile trek at the end of the parade route was tough-it was uphill, and we had no crowds to cheer us on. But amazingly, I wasn't nearly as tired as I had been at age 14. On Jan. 2, when I awoke and took stock of the bodily damage, the only thing that hurt was my jaw. From the start of the parade to the finish, I had grinned from ear to ear.

From 1973 to 1983, I lived and worked on the East Coast.

I went to a lot of small town parades and saw many firefighters showing off their finest uniforms and equipment. I always felt a surge of pride when the bystanders clapped and cheered for their firefighters, but I never really understood the attraction until this January.

On New Year's Day, we were preceded and followed by magnificent floats that each cost $100,000 or more. We could see and hear the public's polite and appreciative reaction to the other floats. But that was no match for the cheers we received. The crowd comprised locals, college football fans from Washington and Indiana, and "snowbirds" who flock to Pasadena each year for the parade and the warm weather. From the center of Colorado Blvd., we saw a sea of faces, 20 deep on the sidewalks and sloping upward as high as 30 feet in temporary grandstands.

As I walked along, I realized how the crowd reflected the region's changing population. Many of those faces were born elsewhere and immigrated to America. Their native cultures had nothing to match the American love affair with the fire service. Still, they smiled broadly and clapped and cheered as our display of firefighting antiquity rolled by.

At 14, I was intent on marching cadence and playing a trumpet. Back then, the whole parade was a blur. But this time my colleagues and I interacted face-to-face with nearly a million people. We had great fun, and I felt honored to have the opportunity to represent the fire service in the granddaddy of all parades.

I'll never again look at a parade without recalling the 2001 Rose Parade. But I'll still feel empathy for those confined by snow and ice on New Year's Day. In exchange, I hope you'll empathize with us the next time we have a brushfire, mudslide or earthquake.

2

Extraordinary People

Who *Was* That Guy?

There comes a time for each of us to be judged. The exact time, place and nature of the proceedings probably have a lot to do with individual spiritual beliefs. Regardless, at the end of life on earth, there is inevitably an inventory of one's accomplishments.

Probably, we will not be judged on how much money we made or saved, how big a house we lived in or the value of the jewelry we wore. Probably, that final judgment will be an appraisal of what our life meant to others.

If that's the case, our friend Harvey D. Grant Jr. easily passed muster when he died of a respiratory disease last January at the age of 58.

Frankly, I don't know anybody who has had more of an impact on the field of rescue than Harvey Grant. Starting in volunteer emergency services at the age of 16, he eventually became fire chief in his hometown of Claymont, Del. But while has activities and contributions in Delaware were many, one state could not contain Harvey's talent and creative energy.

About 20 years ago, Harvey's influence in the fields of rescue and emergency care took a quantum leap. He became the lead author of *Emergency Care*, a textbook that has been used to train

EMS responders worldwide. The book is now in it's sixth edition, and it's estimated that more than 1 ½ million copies have been published. He also wrote or co-authored *Vehicle Rescue, Handbook of Procedures for EMS Personnel*, and numerous magazine and journal articles.

Harvey was instrumental in training some of the first EMS instructors in the United States. He was active with several national organizations, including the International Society of Fire Service Instructors and the International Association of Fire Chiefs (IAFC), and he chaired the ASTM task group that has been developing standards for rescue equipment.

Aside from all the organizational work and meetings, Harvey Grant seemed to enjoy the opportunity to teach and share knowledge most of all. In 1990, for example, Harvey and his company, Rescue Training Associates, made arrangements for the IAFC'S Transportation Emergency Rescue Committee to experiment with extrication techniques on a fleet of *new* cars at the GM proving grounds.

I still remember one of Harvey's finest performances. It was in 1977 in the parking lot of a Los Angeles hotel where a national EMS conference was being held. Harvey and his associates were preparing to demonstrate some vehicle rescue techniques, and I was standing in the crowd with a group of local firefighters.

"What's this all about?" one of the firefighters asked.

"Some volunteer from back East is gonna show us how to cut up cars," answered another sarcastically.

"Why are *we* here?" the first man asked.

"Orders from the chief," their captain replied.

Within 15 minutes, the firefighters were wide-eyed with amazement.

"Geez, did you see *that*?" One exclaimed as Harvey performed magic with a cutting tool.

"Who *is* that guy?" another asked.

I finally spoke up. "His name is Harvey Grant, and he's from back East. He's a friend of mine," I said proudly.

At a memorial service, Harvey's long-time friend and associate Frank Poliafico observed that Harvey was very good at everything he did, including listening. He also commented on Harvey's generosity, giving his time and talent to any and all who needed him. "He really didn't know how to say 'no' to anyone who wanted his help," he said.

Harvey Grant's death has created a void in the rescue community. There may be a few people with the credentials to fill the vacancy, but if they hope to be judged as favorably as Harvey was, they'll need to first recognize and adopt his philosophy of simplicity, hard work and concern for others.

Smooth Operator

"You can usually tell what kind of lover a man is by how he drives a car," the woman with the silky voice announced.

She was a famous madam. She was being interviewed by a radio talk show host late one night as I drove a rented Buick from Stillwater, Okla., to Wichita, Kan. Being a science buff, I turned up the volume.

The talk show host asked the obvious follow-up question. The woman replied that men who drive smoothly and who physically "communicate" with their vehicles have been the most impressive in her experience. Within a moment or two, I caught myself scanning the instrument panel and placing both hands on the steering wheel of the Buick.

Then I thought of John Hanigan. To my knowledge, he wasn't what you might call a "ladies' man." But he could sure drive a fire engine-especially the ones with clutches and manual transmissions.

John was proud to be a guy who understood, maintained, drove, pumped and physically communicated with a fire engine. He didn't strive to be an officer; he was good at what he did and that's more than many people can say about themselves. John also was fun to be around and work with.

"I can drive the engine around the block, put it back in the barn and engage the clutch only once," John said to the crew as they took a Pepsi break one summer afternoon. It was one of those firehouse boasts that just kinda hang in the air, begging somebody to bite-sort of like chumming for shark with chicken entrails.

No reaction.

"Yep," John said, matter-of-factly. "Use the clutch once to get 'er goin', drive out nose-first, go all the way around the block and back 'er in without usin' the clutch again." Everybody knew he was setting them up, but the challenge was too tempting to pass up.

Finally, Danny Mereno couldn't stand it anymore. "All right, damn it. A half gallon a' ice cream says you can't do it." Within minutes, the crew was aboard Engine 15. Mereno was in the front seat, intently watching the clutch pedal.

John started the engine, depressed the clutch pedal and pulled the gearshift into second gear. He smoothly engaged the clutch to get the rig moving. To win the bet, he couldn't use the clutch again, and Mereno knew he'd have to reverse direction to back into the station. You can't do that without using the clutch.

There was no traffic on the residential street, and John left it in second gear till they had completed the turn out of the station. Then, he deftly feathered the engine rpms to neutralize the torque in the gearbox. With the gentlest nudge of the gearshift and his left foot firmly planted on the floor, he disengaged second gear. Then, after the slightest adjustment of rpms, he nudged the lever into third gear as though it were floating in butter.

Around the block they traveled, with John moving the gears between second and third without engaging the clutch. Finally, they were approaching the station. Mereno watched carefully for a trick as John performed another clutchless shift into neutral and allowed the rig to freewheel while traveling parallel to the right-hand curb.

As Engine 15 coasted toward the fire station's driveway, John applied the brakes and made a sharp left turn toward the curbing on the opposite side of the street. As the vehicle approached the curbing, he applied more brake pressure but didn't stop it. As the 16-ton fire engine's front tires simultaneously came in contact with the curb, they absorbed the forward movement and then rebounded, sending the vehicle moving backward. As that happened, John quickly pulled the transmission into reverse-without using the clutch and without grinding a gear.

The rest of the trip was anticlimactic. John backed Engine 15 into the station and nudged the gearshift into neutral without a clutch just before stopping. After purging the air brakes and throwing the master switch, John grinned at the rest of his crew and said, "I'll take rocky road."

Later, he grumbled when they took away his stick shift and gave him a new pumper with an automatic transmission. Our paths didn't cross during those years but others told me that John Hanigan soon learned how to tame a lurching, bucking six-speed automatic. By communicating with his vehicle, sensing the symmetry of constantly changing torque and momentum, and outthinking dozens of little hydraulic valves and electric switches, he gave new meaning to the label "smooth operator."

As I was approaching the Kansas border on I-35, my attention returned to the radio talk show. The host was asking his guest about her most memorable client. "Well, it wasn't one of the famous movie stars or millionaire playboys," she said. "It was a middle-aged bald guy out in L.A. He had big ears, gnarly hands and a gap between his front teeth. As I recall, he was a fireman."

"Hanigan," I shouted into the night. "You son of a gun!"

A Master at His Art

If you've got a copy of *America Burning*, take a look at pages iv and v. The eagle-eyed man pictured in the center died Feb. 28. 1998 Keith E. Klinger was one of the most effective leaders I have ever known.

After he retired from the fire department, Chief Klinger served as a member of the National Commission on Fire Prevention and Control. At the time, 12,000 American lives and more than $11 billion in resources were lost to fire each year. In May 1973, the commission delivered its report (*America Burning*) to President Nixon. For a variety of reasons, our national death toll and fire loss per year has been cut in half since then.

A few years before Chief Klinger retired, Bel Air, California's fire started when combustible vegetation ignited in the Santa Monica Mountains. Within 72 hours, nearly 600 homes had burned, and the mountains looked like a blackened moonscape.

On the first night of the fire, I was driving Assistant Chief Victor Petroff. We were on the move all night long, as the fire moved on a front several miles wide, eating its way through the brush, flaring up and dying down with each change in wind, slope or fuel density. Several times during the night, we met on dusty fire roads with Chief Klinger and his driver.

When we weren't meeting with him, we could hear the boss on the radio, seeking updated information, arranging for meetings with his sector Chiefs, inquiring about the welfare of personnel, and scolding food dispensers to "get over there and take care of those guys." He was 50 years old at the time, but he didn't slow down or sneak off for a nap all night long.

At about 7 a.m. the next day, Chief Klinger held a shift-change meeting with off-going and on-coming chief officers. He was wearing his dark blue work uniform, and it was covered with soot and dust. He was energetic and forceful despite a night without sleep. As the meeting ended, Chief Klinger said to his driver, "Sully, take me downtown," and they drove off in his silver Olds sedan.

The rest of the story was told to me by the late Kenneth Hahn, a member of the Los Angeles County Board of Supervisors (five of the most powerful politicians in California). According to Hahn, the board was having its regular Tuesday morning meeting, and the news was all about the Bel Air Fire and homes lost.

"All of a sudden," Hahn said, "the wooden doors at the back of that big meeting room swung open, and through them marched Chief Klinger. He was covered with soot and dust, and I swear he must have had a fireman out in the lobby with a bellows full of smoke, puffing it through the doorway after the Chief.

"He marched down that aisle like he'd just bought the building," Supervisor Hahn continued. "He wasn't on our official agenda, but he walked right up to the podium and took over the meeting.

"What could we do?" Hahn asked rhetorically. "It seemed the whole county was on fire and the Fire Chief wanted to talk to us. Chief Klinger knew how and when to get attention.

"I noticed he had a folder in his hand," Kenny Hahn remembered. He then recalled how our Chief gave the Board a blow-by-blow report on the battles that were underway in the mountains between Sepulveda Pass and Topanga Canyon. Then, Hahn recalled with a grin, Chief Klinger pulled from the folder a 10-year plan for improvement of fire protection. It called for spending millions of dollars. Again, Hahn asked, "What could we do but vote yes on it?"

The Board of Supervisors adopted Chief Klinger's 10-year plan and provided the money for it, including a fleet of specially designed brush-fire engines and several new fire stations in mountainous areas. Obviously, our Chief had the plan developed long before the Bel Air Fire and had been waiting for the best time to spring it on his elected bosses.

Kenny Hahn and the other supervisors knew they had been set up. But, judging by Hahn's jovial recollections of the event years later, they admired the performance of a Fire Chief who was as good a politician as any of them.

There were many other examples of Keith Klinger's power and effectiveness as a leader. When he retired, the supervisors praised him for the strength and independence he had brought to his position, but they replaced him with someone they'd be able to keep under their thumb.

There aren't many times in life when we get to see a first-class leader doing some of his best work. It was my good fortune to watch and learn from Keith Klinger up close and personal, and I'm one of many who miss him.

Living as a Legacy

A few months ago I heard that *Fire Chief Magazine* would publish a series of articles on the 20 people who most shaped the American fire service in the 20th century. My first thought was, "Why didn't I think of that?" Then I heard they had included me on the list and I haven't been the same since.

In the magazine business, most publishers do their best to pretend that their competitors don't exist. Even though we compete for business, *Fire Chief Magazine's* Publisher Janet Wilmoth and editor Scott Baltic are classy people whose commitment to the fire service and good journalism supercedes petty commercialism.

Fire Chief Magazine calls the series "Legacies." It's dedicated to the late Bill Randleman, *Fire Chief* editor from 1967 to 1990 and one of the finest people I've met.

Alphabetically, the list starts with Francis Brannigan and ends with Lou Witzeman. I've met 11 people on the list and count five of them among my personal friends. One was my boss Keith Klinger-a father figure whose example shaped my career.

I would gladly give up my place on the list to make room for Garry Briese or Al Whitehead. Their success in bringing fire service labor and management closer on some important issues remains one of the more noteworthy achievements in the last century. Others belong on the list, too, such as Rich Marinucci, and I'm sure some names will prove controversial, including mine.

I've run out of wall space for the plaques and awards I've received over the years. Though I feel honored to be on the list, my ego doesn't need further boosting. Beyond the pride of being in such distinguished company, how can we use this listing of influential people to benefit current and future generations?

At this moment there are people among us with a passion for the fire service and an unquenchable desire to challenge the status quo and make things better. What would it take for them to be on a list of the most influential movers and shakers of the first half of the 21st century? Using the examples of people recognized in the *Fire Chief* series, there are some basic requirements for making things happen and getting positive recognition for it.

For example, even in the 1950s, a college education was important if one hoped to become an influential fire-service leader. Ten of the 11 I know on the list received at least an undergraduate degree. Several went on to receive graduate degrees. Almost without exception, they completed or continued their formal education after they joined the fire service. If it was important in the 1950s, it's essential now.

At least two-thirds of the people on the list are published authors. Two good examples: Lloyd Layman and Fred Sheppard. They willingly shared their knowledge, concepts and information with others. They had the ability-either natural or acquired-to put their thoughts into writing and make fire service information educational and sometimes entertaining. They had the self-discipline to plant themselves before a writing tablet, a typewriter or word processor for weeks and months on end to create the books and magazine articles that established them as experts.

At least half the people on the list have been accomplished public speakers. Aside from the ability to stand before a group of colleagues, they mastered the art of verbal communication.

There are some essential talents demonstrated by Alan Brunacini, Ron Coleman, Warren Isman, Keith Klinger and others on the list. For example, genuine fondness for people, thorough knowledge of the fire service, a solid command of the English language, the courage to challenge popular or conventional beliefs and a credible style of presentation.

Unfortunately, there are no women on the list. Maybe that will change in the future. But I do know that more than half the men on the list, including myself, were supported in innumerable ways by strong and understanding spouses. There were times when we passed up overtime shifts in order to teach a class for free. Family vacations and holidays were sacrificed as we completed or continued our education. While writing a book or an article, or preparing a speech, we were unapproachable in our offices or dens. Our wives spent thousands of lonely nights at home while we traveled to far-away places, giving speeches, teaching classes, consulting with colleagues. Nobody earned a spot on *Fire Chief's* "Legacies" list by themselves.

So that's the short list of requirements if you hope for recognition as a fire service leader someday. More than 40 years have passed since I became a firefighter. My first company officer recognized my energy and ambition and put me on the right course. I've experienced tremendous highs and painful setbacks. Whether I deserve it or not, seeing my name on a list with some of the most accomplished people of the 20th century fire service is an honor beyond description. I hope a 21st century firefighter reading this today will be inspired to build a career that can be similarly honored a few decades from now.

3

Fire Service Culture

Friendly Insults

Driving across the country last summer, visiting fire stations and firefighters along the way, I noticed that one of our oldest traditions has survived. It's the practice of joking, kidding, insulting, embarrassing, chiding or otherwise making fun of one another.

In the place where I started my career, it was called "cramming." Other departments, paid and unpaid alike, in different parts of the country have their own labels for this activity. There are times when it has grown out of control, especially water fights and other dangerous practical jokes that cross the line from funny to mean. Still, most of it serves a useful purpose.

Fighting fire and performing rescue operations are group activities. Several people from different backgrounds assemble in a building that resembles a home. (It usually has kitchen, bath and sleeping facilities, plus a big garage.) In the paid fire service, they stay there for long periods of time. In the volunteer service, they assemble in the building for meetings, training, social activities, for stand-by duty, or just to hang out.

When people from the same family get together, there can be stress. When people who are not even related get together in a fire station, there will be even more stress-but most of it will be invisible and subdued. Just getting along with one another can be difficult. But when the alarm sounds, the entire group must function as a disciplined unit in dangerous circumstances under the direction of an officer whose human flaws are known to one and all.

From the moment a newcomer walks into a fire station, the lessons begin. There are some things you can say or do, but there are some limits that aren't written down anywhere. You need to wait a while before you subject someone to a zinger. First, you must be accepted by the group. You'll know you're close to being accepted when you become the target of some friendly insults.

How you react will, in most cases, be the deciding factor. If you can laugh at yourself and if you can tolerate being the butt of someone else's joke, you'll do OK. If you get mad, fight back in anger, sulk or pout, or file a complaint, you'll never find social acceptance in that organization.

The self-appointed guardians of political correctness and all but a few federal judges don't get it. The verbal give-and-take of a typical firehouse would be a hostile workplace in their view. If we lived in a perfect world, probably some of the fire departments I visited last summer would be forced into sensitivity training.

Nationwide, the entire fire service soon will be training for a reality of our times: nuclear, biological and chemical terrorism. Weather phenomena are forecast for next winter that could turn major areas of the country into disaster zones. Last summer, I watched tank cars filled with toxic chemicals traveling on rickety railbeds through little farm towns. What would happen if . . . ?

Who will be the responders of first and last resort when really bad things happen? Local fire departments, that's who. What kind of people will put their own lives on the line to protect the public from the scariest of hazards? It will be those folks who test one another day-to-day with the verbal jousting and practical jokes that are an essential part of firehouse tradition.

A friend of mine who's a master of the art of cramming says there are three reasons for doing it to a colleague. "First, the other person may be one of my best friends and this is my way of letting them know it. Second, the other person needs to modify their standards, habits or behavior and this is how I let them know. Third, I just don't like the other person."

There's a lot of subtlety involved, and you can't regulate subtleties with rules, memos or court orders. There's always the risk of matters spinning out of control, but that, in and of itself, is a test of the maturity of the participants and their supervisors. Most important, it tends to thin the ranks of those who lack the strength of character to work as a reliable member of a team.

Increasingly, firefighters are expected to resolve emergencies that everybody else is running away from. Who else are they gonna call? It's a lot like war. Eventually, small groups of warriors face the enemy in a life-death struggle where teamwork is essential and there's no room for error. Every member of the team needs to know what every other member is made of.

The important firehouse rituals of bonding and testing each other may look like frivolous play to outsiders. Instead, they are time-tested techniques for relieving stress, measuring one another's character and building teamwork. Even as generations come and go, some things never change-and shouldn't.

Your 21st-Century Firefighter

Not long ago, somebody called me an old fart. I'm sure that's happened before, but this was the first time I heard it face-to-face. I knew it was inevitable. I look in the mirror. I can count-birthdays, that is. Recently, I started to use senior citizen cologne (Ben Gay ointment) on my knees after working out. The American Association of Retired Persons somehow got my address, and they send me their magazine, *Modern Maturity*, but I don't read it.

The effect of age on mind and body is inexorable. For some folks, the mind outlasts the body. For others, sadly, the mind goes first. I'm exercising both and hoping they'll work well for another 30 years or so.

In pursuit of mental exercise, I've agreed to write a new textbook to introduce young people to fire and rescue services. In writing the first several chapters, I've tried to imagine how the typical reader will think and act. This will be the person who joins your fire department in the first decade of the 21st century.

He or she will be 18 to 25 years old, with some college education, but still somewhat dependent on mom and dad for housing, major auto repairs, and credit-card bail-outs. This person will have spent many thousands of hours in front of a TV. In households with older siblings or teenage parents, MTV will have been part of our young person's daily entertainment since birth.

At this point, I must explain that I'm trying not to be overly critical of our future firefighter. Old farts criticize those things they can't understand or control. Healthy, inquiring minds-regardless of age-try to understand why things are the way they are and make the most of them.

With that disclaimer on the table, let me continue. Our future firefighter will have precious little experience with teamwork, self-sacrifice, personal organization and respect for authority. It's not necessarily his or her fault. Young people have grown up in the soft, affluent society we created for them. We sold our farms to corporations and won the Cold War so our kids didn't have to bale hay or get drafted.

As the kids grew up, many of us worked multiple jobs so they could have the things we thought were important. Along the way, family meals and table manners were replaced by fast food on the run and notes under refrigerator magnets. Taking a cue from our ingestion of adult beverages and prescription drugs, many of our kids have tried all kinds of chemicals and herbs. Experimentation led to dependence for some.

Many of our kids were sent off to college where their professors really didn't care how they dressed or even whether they showed up for class. Parents prayed their offspring would come home from college as mature, rational adults, finally able to pick up after themselves and speak the king's English. Instead, many learned that in spite of an expensive education, Junior's still a slob who uses the "f" word more frequently than "please" or "thank you."

Again, my sweeping assessment should not be mistaken as criticism of contemporary youth. Although very generally, I've simply pointed to some of the most obvious characteristics of young people, many of whom might want to join you as firefighters. The real question is whether the fire service should change to accommodate those characteristics or whether we should expect individuals to adapt to traditional fire-service standards.

The only legitimate reason for fire departments to exist is to provide the public with emergency services they cannot provide themselves. By their nature, those services must be highly structured within an organization that is competent, well-equipped, properly trained and reliable. Those attributes cannot be achieved without teamwork, self-sacrifice, personal organization and respect for authority.

For about 25 years, the career fire service has cowered under lawsuits, consent decrees, affirmative-action programs and personnel bureaucracies. Much of it was needed to correct an unfortunate history of bias and discrimination. On the other hand, as a consequence of the corrective measures, we now have a generation of officers who seem afraid to do the right thing.

Regardless of generational differences and popular trends, the time has come to take a stand on behalf of the people we serve. Fire and rescue services are complex team functions that must be reliable and skillfully performed. Thus, there are good reasons for fire and rescue personnel to be trained, controlled, clad, equipped and scheduled for the job, rather than for their own personal pleasure or convenience. Young people who have been doing their own thing since age 3 might have no frame of reference for such a disciplined environment. They need and want strong leadership.

For thousands of years, old farts have been predicting that the next generation will be Earth's ruination. For the most part, they've been wrong. Nonetheless, I predict that if we don't re-establish discipline and order in fire departments-career and volunteer alike-the forthcoming generation of firefighters will diminish those attributes that the public depends on most. There are some things more important than "fairness," "equality" and popularity.

Unspoken Rules

I rode to the meeting with a talented young fire officer, somebody I've known and admired for several years. As we drove, he shared with me some of the key issues that would be on the agenda. Nothing really controversial. Officers for the next year would be nominated, a year-end financial report would be presented, and there would be reports on some overdue committee projects.

Our conversation drifted to other topics. I remember thinking, "This guy's got a great future as a fire service leader. He's articulate, he has a command presence, he's not afraid to speak his mind, and he's well-versed on a variety of subjects." It occurred to me that he could make a positive impression in a roomful of bankers, lawyers, doctors or business leaders.

At the meeting, I saw another person emerge. My friend chaired the meeting, and he opened it with a shy and stumbling apology for being unfamiliar with parliamentary procedure. "We can have committee reports, or however you guys want to do it is OK with me," he said in a very submissive way.

When it came time for the financial report, the treasurer handed out copies of a balance sheet he had prepared. "I'm not too familiar with accounting," he said, "but I'll try to answer any questions." I happened to know that the treasurer had a very successful business, in addition to his work with the fire department. I knew he could not have succeeded in his business without a solid working knowledge of accepted accounting principles.

What was going on here? My friend, the chairman of the meeting, was intentionally hiding his talents and skills. The treasurer of the organization was playing dumb. Why?

Whether paid or unpaid, the fire service consists of people who must function harmoniously in groups. Individuals from different backgrounds and varying levels of talent come together for long periods of time in a setting that resembles a home. They must get along with each other because the next alarm could thrust the entire group into a situation of great jeopardy. They may find themselves depending on each other in the face of life-threatening risks.

Over the decades, patterns of behavior have emerged to assure harmony among firefighters-or, at least, to prevent conflict. For veterans, most of those behaviors are instinctive. For newcomers, the proper attitudes and behaviors are learned quickly or the individual is more or less banished from the group.

Let's face it. The solidarity among firefighters is one of our greatest strengths-and a source of mystery (and even jealousy and resentment) to some "outsiders." But any strength, when taken to an extreme, becomes a weakness.

In many cases, we have served the fire service culture of solidarity by "dumbing down" to the level of the lowest common denominator. My friend has enough talent to chair a session of the United Nations Security Council. Yet, in a small group of fellow firefighters, he pretended to be unskilled at parliamentary procedure. In his fire department's culture, one is expected to avoid embarrassing or showing up the least skilled member of the group, especially if that person outranks you.

Varying degrees of this phenomenon occur in most North American fire departments. Watch for the signs and signals in your own department, or in yourself. Is there pressure to not stand out? Have you felt a need to speak or act less smart or well-informed than you really are? Have you seen others pay a price for being too quick with the right answers or for being too sure of themselves? Anthropologists would say that they've broken the unspoken rules of group socialization.

It's worked pretty well for more than 200 years. The group that suppresses individuality and achieves harmony in routine circumstances usually functions well in emergencies. But for most of our fire service history, the enemy (fire) has been dangerous but dumb, and reasonably predictable.

The fire service of today has some new enemies. Some are politicians or public administrators who seek change for its own sake. Some are entrepreneurs who hope to make a profit from public safety. Others are molders of public opinion with an axe to grind. Though most of these enemies are simply ill-informed or misguided, they are nonetheless smart and unpredictable-thus dangerous. They trivialize the fire problem and try to reduce the resources we need to prevent and suppress fires.

How can we, the fire service, effectively stand up to our enemies while we handicap ourselves with the unspoken rules of group socialization? Pit a group of smart, unrestrained people against a group that feels compelled to think, act and speak at the level of the lowest common denominator, and then place a bet on the likely winner. Who will it be?

Watch for the signs and signals in your own organization. Next time someone slips up and makes a profoundly intelligent statement, watch the rest of the group pounce on it with a vengeance. Next time someone volunteers for a task, watch for others in the group to criticize the outcome, whether it's good or bad. Watch and listen to those who are natural leaders (regardless of rank). Do they restrain their leadership instincts in deference to those with less talent?

Can we maintain harmony while giving our members the liberty of thinking, talking, acting and performing to the full extent of their abilities? Is the practice of group socialization (dumbing down to the level of the lowest common denominator) necessary to maintain harmony in a fire company or department? Does this practice become self-fulfilling-driving off or breaking the spirit of the more talented people while fostering mediocrity?

Probably, your answers to these questions depend on the culture of your organization and how well you fit into it. The answers aren't as important as the questions. Until and unless we feel free to be our best among each other, and to show it, we won't be competitive in the world that now confronts us.

Heroes and Hyperbole

As a group of NASA scientists met, they discussed the potential fate of their latest multimillion dollar effort to land a robot on Mars. One of them said, "We'll either be heroes or zeros." There's that word again-"hero." It gets used a lot these days, inappropriately as often as not. Some examples:

• At the annual dinner of an association of fire department boards of directors, a prominent politician gave the after-dinner speech. Apparently, thinking he was talking to a room full of firefighters, the politician said, "To me, and the people you serve, you're all heroes." The audience applauded heartily.

• A 17-foot aluminum boat containing 14 people departed Cuba en route to Florida. The boat sank and most of its occupants vanished, including the mother of a small boy. The boy clutched an inflated innertube and floated for hours until some American fishermen plucked him from the sea. News reports called the boy's struggle for survival "heroic."

In Greek mythology, Hero was a priestess of Aphrodite. A guy named Leander was in love with Hero. Every night he would swim across the Dardanelles, a four-mile-wide strait, to visit her. When she found Leander drowned, Hero drowned herself and thus became famous.

Does that mean the NASA scientists will drown themselves because their robot crashed and doesn't work? How did we get from the myth of a suicidal priestess to a roomful of out-of-shape old men gleefully accepting the label "hero"? If the little Cuban boy had followed the mythical Hero's example, he would have traded his innertube for a watery grave in grief over his mother's drowning.

Hyperbole (high-PUR-buh-lee) is exaggeration for effect. Hyperbolic statements are not meant to be taken literally. Examples in this column's context are "We're the greatest" and "We're No. 1!" As a society greatly influenced by competitive media and sports, we're constantly bombarded by hyperbole. You've probably heard the shorter form of the word-hype.

Unfortunately, hyperbole has crept into the world of the fire and rescue service, especially the use of the word "hero." There's no rule that says myths can't evolve and adapt with time, and that's what happened in the 3,500 years since Leander drowned en route to the warm embrace of his lover. The question is whether overuse of the term hero will rob it of its commonly accepted meaning.

Regardless of its roots in Greek mythology, "hero" came to represent a person who performed an extremely difficult or dangerous act to help or save another person or persons. Many heroes have lost their lives in acts of heroism. Two world wars and the Korean and Vietnam wars influenced the meaning of the term for Americans. Battlefield reports included stories of men who threw themselves on hand grenades to save their fellow soldiers from the blast.

The Russians probably had the greatest role in diminishing the modern meaning of heroism. During 70 years of communist rule, Hero of the Soviet Union awards were granted by the thousands. Presumably, they started out as tributes for courage on the battlefield. By 1989, the Soviet hero awards were issued to mediocre bureaucrats and ruthless enforcers of the Kremlin's rules. Today in Russia, you can't trade one for a loaf of bread.

A visit to the Internet reveals some of the more recent uses of the word. For example, an off-duty police officer used the Heimlich maneuver on a choking child in a restaurant and received a heroism award from a community group. That's a long way from the soldier who sacrificed himself on a grenade. Public-safety personnel are trained to react appropriately when confronted by a person choking. Is that really an act of heroism? What if he was on duty?

We've been trained to enter burning buildings, rescue trapped people and extinguish fires. Is it an act of heroism? Sure, it's dangerous, but a lot of jobs are dangerous. Does that make the people who do those jobs heroes?

What about a firefighter who dies while fighting a fire? Is that firefighter a hero? What if the firefighter didn't die, but was badly injured? What if the injury or death was due to a foolish error or a violation of safety standards?

I don't mean to diminish the importance or the inherent dangers of firefighting and other emergency services. But it's not wise to overstate those dangers or to give hero awards to people who probably aren't heroes in the traditional sense. It leads to hyperbole, and hyperbole could lead a cynical public to equate the fire service with car dealers.

Occasionally, somebody does something for others that's truly extraordinary-a selfless act, above and beyond the call of duty, and involving great personal danger with no expectation of special recognition or reward. Let's save the hero label for those occasions. Let's discourage frivolous use of the word before it becomes as mythical as the priestess of Aphrodite.

4

California Firestorms

Fire in the Elfin Forest

In October1991, firefighters in the hilly residential areas east of the San Francisco Bay fought a deadly and destructive natural phenomenon. Investigators reported that the Oakland Hills fire was started by people who were burning tree trimmings. But the forces that turned that "controlled burn" into a billion-dollar conflagration were the almost-predictable work of nature.

If you live and work in Minnesota, Massachusetts, Maine or Missouri, it's probably hard to understand how a vegetation fire can spread so easily to hundreds of homes. And even if you've experienced range fires in the Dakotas or Kansas or the fires that ravage the underbrush in Florida, the Carolinas or the Jersey Pine Barrens, you've probably marveled at the TV coverage of California's firestorms.

Normally, weather in North America moves from west to east. Sometimes, however-usually between September and December-a quirk occurs over the southwestern states. High pressure develops over Utah, Nevada and Arizona at the same time that low pressure develops over the Pacific Ocean near California. This causes a mass movement of air from east to west.

As air moves toward the west, it crosses parched deserts, and moisture is sucked from it as it approaches the Pacific mountain ranges. These mountains form a barrier the air must cross in its pursuit of the low pressure over the ocean. The rivers of warmed air are compressed as they crest the mountains, causing them to speed up as they flow down the coastal canyons.

These hot, down-slope winds have acquired the label "Santa Ana." It's unclear how they got the name. Some say the Chumash Indians called them the winds of the devil, that white men changed that to "satan winds," which later were referred to as "satanta winds" and, still later, "Santa Ana." Another explanation is that they were named after Santa Ana Canyon, where they usually blow first and worst.

The western slopes of the Pacific ranges are primarily covered with dense, dry vegetation that has been called the "elfin forest." Generically referred to as chapparal, it includes chemise, buckbrush, cyanothis, sage, sumac and manzanita. Living in dry, rocky soil, these hardy species rarely grow more than 20 feet tall and are capable of surviving long periods without rain. Added to this shrubbery mix approximately 100 years ago was a tough, oily, drought-resistant Australian import, the eucalyptus.

The Oakland fire occurred about a month short of the 30th anniversary of the infamous Bel Air, Calif., fire. On the morning that inferno started, winds at the top of Stone Canyon were blowing in excess of 50 mph, humidity was less than 5 percent, and the air temperature was nearly 90 F-at 0800 hours.

Most vegetation wilts and dies when subjected to such extreme conditions for more than a few hours. However, for millions of years, the native plant life of the Pacific ranges has been evolving and has developed a protective response. Cued by nature, the bushes, shrubs and stunted trees of the elfin forest exude an oily substance that coats the leaves and branches, sealing in the precious moisture that would otherwise be leached out by the hot, dry winds.

The problem is, the oily substance burns quite readily in those atmospheric conditions. One study that was conducted a few years ago found that 20 acres of this vegetative fuel, all burning at once, can produce as much heat as the atomic bomb that leveled Hiroshima. Typically, giant mushroom-shaped clouds of black and gray smoke rise 10,000 feet or more before they are swept out over the ocean.

It's all part of nature's plan. Many of the species in the elfin forest cannot propagate without the help of periodic fires. Still others will be choked by their own dead underbrush unless there is a fire every 20 to 40 years. But nature didn't count on people building their houses in the middle of it all-with wood-shingle roofs.

Although wooden roofs make houses more vulnerable, veteran firefighters will tell you that many houses burn from the inside out when they are caught in a typical brush fire. Once the firestorm creates its own winds to supply oxygen to fire, it picks up burning debris and carries it forward, starting spot fires ahead of the main fire. When large pieces of burning debris strike and break the windows of a structure, they usually start an interior fire.

The people who fought the Oakland fires and rescued residents from the onslaught deserve our utmost respect. Tackling a rapidly moving and dangerous enemy, in air that's unfit to breathe and filled with burning cinders, with hot wind strong enough to knock a person down and roaring loud enough to drown out the sound of radio traffic-and working for 12 hours or more without a break-may be the ultimate challenge in emergency services.

Incident command, training and experience, tactics and strategy, good equipment, adequate water and airborne support, physically fit firefighters and logistical support all contribute to the effort to manage vegetation fires at the urban-wildland interface. But the weather always determines when and where the fire will be extinguished. And, just to make sure things don't get too badly out-of-hand, Mother Nature constructed a firebreak to halt the progress of even the wildest of wildfires. It's called the Pacific Ocean.

Surfing With The Devil

Watching TV reports of the recent fires in Southern California produced a flood of memories for me. Especially when a fire jumped a ridge on the edge of the San Fernando Valley and raced through Topanga Canyon toward the ocean.

Twenty-four years earlier, I was the fire captain on duty at Station 69 in Topanga Canyon. The Santa Anas were blowing, and the air was pungent with the fragrance of native vegetation as it protects itself against the hot, dry winds. Our fire company consisted of five people, a pumper and two small patrol trucks.

We all knew the weather conditions were ripe for a fire, so early in the day we deployed both patrol units. We roamed the public roads throughout our 100-aquare-mile area, making ourselves visible, scaring off would-be arsonists and watching for smoke.

I was in Patrol 69 around noon when we received an alarm: "Brush fire reported in Woodland Hills north of Topanga Canyon Boulevard."

Looking in the direction, I saw the header, flipped on the lights and siren and headed toward it. Engine 69 was responding from the station, and Patrol 269 was en route from Old Topanga Canyon.

As I wrestled the small truck through the road's twists and turns, I was thinking of the advice of old-timers who had fought a half-dozen fires in the same terrain. The only way to keep a fire out of Topanga is to stop it at the ridge that separates Woodland Hills from the canyon, they had said. But nobody had ever been able to stop a wind-driven fire at the ridge. I wanted us to be the first.

Every year, a fire department bull-dozer clears a fuel break along the ridge, and a dirt fire road passes through the middle of the cleared area. I pulled the patrol truck onto the fire road and drove a quarter-mile to a saddle where I could look down on the fire. The wind had died down, and the smoke was rising straight up.

A few minutes later, Engine 69 arrived on scene. "We've got a chance of stopping this thing here at the ridge," I explained to the crew. "If the wind doesn't pick up."

My plan was to backfire from the ridge toward the fire. That way, when the fire made its run to the top, it would run out of fuel before gaining the momentum necessary to cross the fuel break.

We spaced ourselves about a hundred years apart and began lighting backfires. The brush burned eagerly, and the backfires began to grow together.

Just then, the hot wind picked up and started to blow in gusts of 50 mph or more. About the same time, the heat from the main fire and our backfires merged to produce a kind of flashover.

Spontaneously, we started running for our vehicles-but we couldn't run fast enough. I had the sensation of being inside the curl of a giant ocean wave. But the substance of the curl was hot beyond description and was filled with biting smoke and red-hot embers.

It was like surfing in hell. As we ran, it was impossible to see or breathe. The embers were like a swarm of angry bees, finding their way into gloves, boots, collars and pant legs. By the time we arrived at our pumper, the engine had died for lack of oxygen. We all rushed to the patrol truck and crowded into the cab. Before I could close the windwing, a thousand hot embers blew in after us.

In two or three minutes, the worst was over, and we re-emerged into the smoke and embers to extinguish fires that had started in the pumper's upholstery, hosebed and storage bins. At the same time, I reported to incoming units that the fire had slopped over the ridge and was heading into Topanga Canyon.

Two days later, the fire was contained-after the weather changed and moist ocean air replaced the Santa Anas. During those two days, my thoughts were dominated by remorse. In the quest for personal achievement, I had placed my crew in a position of unacceptable risk.

In the years following that fire, the brush grew back, as it has for tens of thousands of years. And now it has burned again, as it must to propagate.

The most to be gained from that frightening episode is a lesson I am compelled to share with others who are entrusted with the lives and welfare of emergency services personnel.

In pursuit of a personal challenge, I placed my crew in jeopardy. They survived and forgave me, but I have never forgiven myself. The brush grew back, but dead firefighters cannot be replaced. Regardless of our emergency service environment, let that be a lesson to all of us.

The Ultimate Challenge

Instead of eating lunch, I went for a swim. Later, drying off on the pool deck in the warm sun, I noticed a slight breeze from the east. It was October 21, humidity was 14 percent, and the infamous "Santa Ana" winds were stirring.

Later, as I was leaving the gym, I scanned the horizon for smoke. A single pillar of black appeared to the east, in the direction of the rural community of Harmony Grove. The color indicated heavy fuel but it was rising straight up; the wind wasn't a factor at the moment.

I thought of the volunteer firefighters who would be first-due. For some, it would be their first big fire. With some luck, good leadership, pinpoint waterdrops and calm winds, they should be able to hold it to two or three acres. I drove back to the office.

About 3 p.m., I looked out a window to the east. The horizon was almost entirely black. The smoke was blowing west, out over the ocean. The eucalyptus trees outside were waving in the wind. It occurred to me that this one could be disastrous.

The area where the fire was burning is shaped something like a huge, irregular bowl, covered with native combustible vegetation. Since prehistoric times, a creek has been carving a depression that allows the bowl to drain west. As it flows toward the ocean, the creek has etched a deep, mile-wide cleft in the middle of the La Costa section of Carlsbad, Calif. It's called Box Canyon; it's been home to all manner of native wildlife; and its vegetation hadn't burned in more than 50 years.

On the afternoon of October 21, the "devil winds" turned the path of San Marcos Creek into a horizontal flue, blowing superheated air and sparks from the Harmony Grove fire into Box Canyon. The canyon exploded in the fashion of an A-bomb, vaporizing its botanical and zoological contents. As roiling fireballs rose out of the canyon, an airborne slurry of embers poured onto the roofs of nearby homes.

By the time this happened, Carlsbad's entire roster of career firefighters had been recalled, and they were assisted by mutual aid strike teams from near and far. None of those firefighters will ever forget that afternoon and evening, but few will ever find the words to adequately describe what they endured.

I've tried in the past to paint an accurate word picture of this phenomenon. For example, *"Tackling a rapidly moving and dangerous enemy, in air that's unfit to breathe and filled with burning cinders, with hot wind strong enough to knock a person down and roaring loud enough to drown out the sound of radio traffic-and working for 12 hours or more without a break-may be the ultimate challenge in emergency services."* [1]

Another time, in admitting to a tactical error, *I described the fire that swept over my crew and me. "I had the sensation of being inside the curl of a giant ocean wave. But the substance of that curl was hot beyond description and was filled with biting smoke and red-hot embers. As we ran, it was impossible to see or breathe. The embers were like a swarm of angry bees, finding their way into gloves, boots, collars and pant legs."* [2]

On the night of October 21, I stayed up late, listening to a scanner as my home-town fire department ran its biggest fire ever with a smooth-as-silk incident command system. More than once, I got a lump in my throat as I remembered the chaos of big fires in the days before ICS. A few days later, I toured the streets that sit on the edges of Box Canyon. Fifty-four luxury homes had burned to the ground, stark evidence of the hazards of wood shingle roofs.

A closer look told a bigger story, however. Generally, it's felt that no effective fire suppression can occur in the middle of a firestorm. But, right on the edge of that canyon, houses with wood-shingle roofs had been saved. Roof fires had been stopped by firefighters who couldn't get a breath of clean air as they struggled to keep their footing on slippery shingles in winds strong enough to bend a hose stream.

By the time I got there, the burned areas of numerous wood roofs were covered with plastic sheeting. I hoped that the homeowners and their insurers fully appreciated how and why those homes had suffered only the partial loss of their roofs. They were the beneficiaries of extraordinary performances, if not downright heroism.

Several years ago, my wife and I had a home on the edge of Box Canyon. The canyon was full of life and, at night, we would hear nocturnal wildlife engaged in the rituals of feeding, breeding and protecting territory. Daytime, we enjoyed the birds as they ventured from their natural sanctuary to the fringes of our world. In the winter, after rainstorms, we could hear water rushing over rocky falls deep in the canyon.

Today, Box Canyon is a desolate black moonscape. In three to four months, it will be covered by the green fuzz of new vegetation. In five years, it will be repopulated by wildlife. In another generation, it will burn again. For the sake of those who reside on the edge of the canyon at that time I have two wishes.

I wish they will have sense enough to roof their homes with non-combustible materials, and I wish for them to be served by firefighters who are as fit, skillful and courageous as those who were there on October 21, 1996.

References

1. *"Fire in the Elfin Forest," Rescue, January/February 1992.*
2. *"Surfing with the Devil," Rescue, January/February 1994.*

5

When Things Go Wrong

The Cost of Chaos

A few weeks ago, I spent a long Saturday in a hotel room in an Atlantic Coast state. My business in the area didn't finish until Friday evening, and, for some strange reason, the air fare back to the West Coast is $500 cheaper if you stay through Saturday night. So there I sat, reading everything I could get my hands on, including a local weekly newspaper.

The headline "Rescuers Deal With a Failure" caught my eye. The first paragraph explained that two days after an 18-year-old-youth died under a bridge, investigators were still trying to figure out who did what at the scene. The second paragraph said that the problems created by crowds and confusion were compounded by the fact that there may have been no clear commander coordinating the efforts of the ten emergency response teams at the scene.

Quite accidentally, I had stumbled onto a story that illustrates a situation that should no longer exist in emergency services. Too many resources in an emergency can be worse than not enough. And emergency resources operating without the coordination of a single, undisputed commander often make matters worse. Too often, an uncontrolled rescue operation becomes deadly for the rescuers themselves.

Reporters for small-town newspapers are often just getting started in the journalism business. Unfortunately, their reporting tends to show the lack of experience. The writer of the rescue article left the readers hanging: After mentioning confusion at the rescue scene and the lack of a clear command structure, he switched gears and wrote the rest of the article about the anguish the rescuers were feeling.

Still, I could read between the lines. The driver of a small car had lost control while crossing a 12-foot-deep canal on a narrow bridge and the car plunged into the water. The 16-year-old female driver got out of the car and swam to safety. The young man did not surface from the brackish water.

According to the newspaper, at least 100 people got involved in the rescue effort. To get a better picture of the situation, I left the hotel room and drove a rental car to the bridge where the rescue had occurred. There was no way that more than a hundred people could have been deployed safely in that terrain. In fact, more than 20 rescuers would have been pushing safety and common sense to the limits.

The basic problem is familiar to most of you: A rescue incident occurs at the borderline between jurisdictions and everybody responds. When the emergency gets toned out, members of neighboring rescue organizations respond without being requested. Due to organizational pride and independence, no single organization or commander takes clear-cut authority over the scene. So, almost everybody ends up freelancing.

Public expectations about what rescuers can and should do have been unreasonably elevated. More and more often, when rescuers arrive at an emergency scene, citizens or reporters scream at them to do things that are not smart to do. This is all the more reason for each emergency to have a single commander who will take control and who can order the public and the media away from the working area.

The well-trained incident commander must conduct a risk-benefit analysis at every step of managing the emergency.

Questions must be considered, such as: How long has the victim been submerged? What is the likelihood that victim could be resuscitated even if located and retrieved immediately after rescuers arrive? Is the water cold enough to trigger the mammalian diving reflex? How many rescuers should be deployed at one time? Are the rescuers properly trained, physically fit and adequately equipped? What is the risk that they too will become victims?

This is not a job for wimps or scatterbrains. The incident commander is likely to be criticized, no matter how the rescue unfolds. With hordes of sidewalk superintendents, and with emotions controlling many people's minds and mouths, everyone will have an opinion on how it should be done. So be it. But there should never be a question as to whether there is a command structure, and who is in charge.

As I stood on that flimsy bridge on an overcast Saturday, I looked down into the murky water of the canal. Imagining a hundred people or more frantically trying to locate the submerged victim brought back images of rescues turned even more tragic.

We've all seen the chilling pictures of rescuers trapped in the eddies of a low-head dam. California's Convict Lake tragedy was another awful reminder of the need for incident command. Rescues that are dominated by the emotions of freelance rescuers sometimes save a victim; more often, they fail to save the victim, while injuring or killing one or more of the rescuers.

Whether we are volunteers or career rescuers, whether we work in urban, suburban or rural areas, whether we work in fire services or independent rescue services, we must put incident command at the top of our agenda. By its nature, rescue will always be dangerous. But there is no excuse for a rescue operation to become even more dangerous simply because it lacks adequate organization and command.

A Tragedy of Errors

Pete and Cindy were on a Saturday drive when they came across a head-on collision on the outskirts of a suburban city. Pete is a fire officer and Cindy is an EMT. A Chevy Caprice had crossed the center line into the path of a Ford Escort carrying a man, his wife and their two young sons.

Pete commandeered the cellular phone in a spectator's Mercedes while Cindy began to assess the victims. The two boys in the back seat of the Escort seemed to be in the most serious condition. The doors were jammed. Pete knocked out the windows at the rear and right rear, crawled up on the deck lid and leaned through the window opening until he could reach one of the boys. Cindy was assessing the other child through the right rear window opening.

Pete felt for the boy's pulse and it seemed too fast. The boy was unconscious and his skin looked ashen. In the distance a siren could be heard. Belly down on the trunk of the wrecked car, with pieces of tempered glass pressing through this thin shirt, Pete held the 10-year-old's head in a neutral position and tried to monitor his breathing.

Later, Pete told me that he had prayed for the boy to live.

"I've never been very religious," he said. "But I could feel a life slipping away between my two hands. I prayed to God for him to live until the medics could get there. I kept saying, 'Give him a chance, God, please give him a chance'."

The siren got closer and a police cruiser finally arrived. The police officer immediately started directing traffic. Ten minutes had passed since Pete and Cindy had arrived on scene. Pete's arms were cramping as he continued to hold traction on the boy's head and neck. Cindy's pink jumpsuit had blood on it that trickled from the inside of her upper arm where she had snagged some glass while working through the window opening.

Another siren approached, accompanied by the sounds of a diesel engine and jake brake. It was a fire engine-a three-person fire engine. The fire captain made his radio report and climbed down off the rig. He was wearing bunker pants and boots, a short-sleeved shirt, no gloves, no helmet, no eye protection and had no tool in hand.

The captain worked his way around the wreckage till be encountered Pete, who suggested they get busy removing the roof of the Escort. The officer replied that his rig didn't have any extrication equipment but that he would radio for a truck company. Meanwhile, a paramedic ambulance with a two-person crew arrived.

Another 10 minutes passed before the Truck Company and a chief officer arrived. During that 10 minutes, the paramedics and firefighters were limited in what they could do for the trapped accident victims. Two firefighters took over for Pete and Cindy. One of the kids had vomited and Pete had tried to maintain traction while clearing the boy's mouth. He noticed there was blood in the vomit.

Even after the chief officer arrived, no command post was established. In fact, there seemed to be no command of any kind. The truck company crew dismounted in varying stages of dress-none of them ready to go to work. Their first official action was to wander around the cars. The chief got on his radio and called for two tow trucks.

It was a firefighter who finally took some control over the situation. He instructed two other firefighters to get the hydraulic equipment and some cribbing off the truck. According to Pete, it took 46 minutes to get the roof off the Escort.

It was clear that the crew had not drilled or performed with their equipment regularly. They had no predetermined plan of action. They would all work on cutting a door pillar, or they would all work to pry a door open until they all got frustrated, and then they would start another operation. The power unit for their hydraulic equipment failed repeatedly, as thought it were trying to run on old or dirty fuel.

By the time the roof of the car was removed, it was nearly dark. It had been an hour since the first fire company had arrived on scene. Some portable lights had been set up, casting long shadows across the work area and making the patients' pale skin look even more pale.

As the 10-year-old was lifted from the crushed vehicle, his shallow breathing ceased and he gasped. The medics did a quick check, started CPR, loaded him into their ambulance and headed for the nearest hospital. The boy did not survive.

Would he have survived if the rescuers had been better equipped and prepared? We'll never know. Did he have a right to a more skilled, efficient and better-equipped rescue effort? Absolutely. There is no valid excuse for anything less.

Internal Strife

In my travels visiting with you and your colleagues, I often ask, "How's it going?" or "How ya doin'?" Usually, the answer is "fine," "good," "OK" or "terrific." After a few cups of coffee and an hour or more of conversation, I usually ask the question again, and the truth begins to emerge.

It's not a matter of being nosy or looking for trouble. I'm trying to make sure FireRescue Magazine lives up to its motto: "Read it today, use it tomorrow." We need to know what you're dealing with before we can offer advice or information about how to deal with it. Besides, when people decide you really care, most are glad to share the details of how they really are "doin'."

In the past two years, I've heard a recurring theme. Internal strife among members of fire departments has become epidemic.

Although it occurs in both career and volunteer departments, it seems pronounced among volunteers. Increasingly, people seem to have difficulty subduing their personal interests to achieve mutual goals.

Again and again, I've heard the stories of projects, assignments, fund-raising campaigns, or special events that ended in bitter conflict among those who volunteered to organize or assist.

Increasingly, members of committees compete for the personal recognition (but don't want to be responsible for things that go wrong). In most cases, one or more people decline a formal leadership position, but work behind the scenes to exercise negative leadership, pitting people against each other by planting and fostering criticism and suspicion.

Hearing stories and living through the experience are two different things. Earlier this year, I was asked to provide technical advice, financial guarantees and operating cash for a national event being put together by a loosely organized group of volunteers. Let's call it the "Big Event."

It sounded like a great idea and, before I even mentioned it to my wife, I was on the hook for about $20,000.

The person who talked me into that commitment promptly took charge. She called often for advice, followed my recommendations, kept me informed and pursued the details with determination. Occasionally, she would share with me some minor disputes that popped up with members of the organizing committee.

I didn't have the time or patience to deal with petty bickering, but I should have taken the time and nipped it in the bud.

The Big Event occurred, and it was a huge success. Everybody who helped plan and present the event could take pride in its success. I even got my money back.

Although most attendees never knew it, the Big Event was marred by conflict among the very people who made it a success. Several times over three days I was confronted by breathless, wide-eyed (or tearful) reports of pending crisis, or tattletale renditions of what other people said or didn't say, did or didn't do.

I've spent most of my life with firefighters, most of whom subdue their personal interests when teamwork is essential to getting the job done. They may have differences, but they wait until the right time and place to discuss and resolve them. I'm not very gentle with people who get into petty disputes on the fireground.

In the middle of the Big Event, when hundreds of people were having the time of their lives, some of the hardest working of the volunteers lost their perspective. Something resembling a mutiny started to occur (against the person I had empowered and entrusted). Instinctively, my demeanor became tactless and to the point. The mutiny collapsed, the attendees continued to enjoy themselves, and I was reviled by some of the would-be mutineers as an insensitive ingrate. If I'd been a volunteer fire chief and if they'd been members, my hopes for re-election would be iffy.

In the aftermath, I've thought many times about the message I've been hearing from many of you. People seem unable to get things done in groups without internal strife and conflict. Some would rather fight than win. Others have no concept of organizational dynamics. Almost every organization has people who reserve the opportunity to stand back and watch others volunteer, then subvert or criticize the effort from a safe distance.

Few Americans under the age of 35 have had military training. People who've grown up in permissive environments may have little experience with disciplined behavior in group endeavors. With that in mind, here are a few ground rules that might be announced whenever somebody proposes a project, campaign or event:

• Power follows money. If you really want to be in charge, find the money to make it happen and then accept responsibility for the money and the outcome.

• There can only be one boss at a time. To really make things happen, one person should be selected to be the boss, authority should be commensurate with responsibility and the person selected should be protected from snipers.

• Pick the proper time and place to raise questions and file complaints, and don't get emotional (tears kill credibility).

• Join in or shut up. If you have a chance to participate and don't, you have forfeited the right to intervene or complain.

• Virtue is its own reward. The only kind of praise that's worth a damn is that which you didn't seek or expect.

Nightmares on Main Streets

You know you're an activist if you get excited by the opportunity to influence change. Activists are energized by visions of how things can be. They have little patience with people who say, "We tried that once, and it didn't work," or "That may work in some places, but we're different."

The activist's dream is to have his or her ideas warmly greeted and implemented without alteration. As the dream continues, the idea or concept works like a charm and everybody credits the activist for making things better. In the activist's nightmare, the idea or concept is flatly rejected but he or she fights long and hard for acceptance. Eventually, the dream gets implemented, but the people who could make it work do a bad job.

I'm an activist, and I've had a few dreams come true-but I've had a lot more nightmares. One of those nightmares slaps me in the face when I visit some of America's biggest cities.

The riots and arson fires of the 1960s taught us a lot about commanding incidents and fighting fires. As those old buildings burned, I realized an era was ending. The supply of old buildings would ultimately dwindle and be replaced by vacant lots or new structures with built-in fire protection. Except in a few urban areas, ours would be the last generation to fight a working fire almost every duty shift.

At the time, career firefighters ranked economically within the lower middle class. Many of us had to work extra jobs to support our families. My dream was to see us elevated to professional status with salaries and fringe benefits to match. I ran for office in my union to help make that happen. The tide began to shift our way in the 1970s but, just over the horizon was the ominous question of productivity.

Many of my colleagues never worried about the future, but I knew that working fires would become rare. I knew we could never maintain our staffing and improved salaries and benefits unless we were more productive. Some city managers had plans to merge us with the cops, make us wax floors in city hall or mow the lawns in city parks. Meanwhile, there was a glaring need that we could satisfy while enhancing our status as emergency professionals.

When people were injured or became ill 30 years ago, there was a deadly gap between their call for help and the arrival of an ambulance. Meanwhile, in many cases, firefighters sat on a bench in front of their station and watched the ambulance go by on its way to a heart attack or an auto crash a block away.

I shared a dream with other activists. We believed that fire companies could perform a valuable function as medical first responders. They could save lives and protect people against further injury. They could bring calm and order to the scenes of medical emergencies. They could justify the cost of full-time, fully staffed career fire companies. They would better meet the public's expectations for productivity.

For years, we tried to sell the concept. At first, most chiefs and many firefighters blew it off as unrelated to the mission of the fire service. They didn't understand that achieving greater productivity, while keeping the fire company together in other forms of emergency work, could be used to justify full staffing. There's no substitute for fully staffed fire companies when the big fire happens-however rarely. That staffing won't be there unless its cost can be justified day in and day out.

The nightmares occur frequently when I witness a medical emergency in some of America's big cities. Typically, an engine company arrives with the siren still cranked up. Occasionally, there is a ceremonial air horn blast as the rig stops-as if to jolt the patient into ventricular fibrillation. What follows is a ritual of casual indifference, hands-in-the-pockets nonchalance, vague simulations of patient assessment and care and active listening for the sound of an ambulance.

The worst example I've seen happened recently. A young man had suffered a seizure on a downtown street. I stopped to see if I could help. With another bystander, I checked the victim's breathing and pulse, tried to protect his airway and comfort him.

Very soon, a fire engine arrived and three guys slowly got off the rig. One knelt down to ask a few questions, but never touched the victim. A second guy leaned against the rig and clipped his fingernails. The third guy never looked at the victim, but walked over to check out the wares of a nearby sidewalk vendor. The ambulance arrived a few minutes later. Immediately, the fire crew got on their rig without even talking to the ambulance crew. As the engine left, its exhaust pipe covered the entire scene with a cloud of diesel smoke.

This isn't brain surgery. It's a matter of common decency, professional behavior and public appearances. The dream has been implemented, but some of the people who can make it work are doing a bad job. That's a nightmare.

6

The Ride of My Life

The Reincarnation of Rescue 11

If you're like most rescuers I've known, you appreciate things that are mechanical tools, equipment, machines, rescue vehicles. In fact, you probably have a favorite rescue vehicle. It may be one that you helped design, or maybe it was the first one you ever worked on.

The most memorable part of my first rescue call was responding to the scene. My partner was a guy with 18-inch biceps and a lead foot. Our rig was a '47 Ford half-ton panel truck. We entered the dogleg curve on El Molino Avenue with the little flathead V-8 wound tight in second gear (about 40 mph). The weight of the truck and our rescue tools shifted, and the truck leaned heavily first in one direction and then in the other.

My partner wrestled with the steering wheel and let out a "yahoo" in the middle of the turn, about the time I was wondering whether we would survive the ride. A half-mile farther and we approached the busy intersection at Lincoln Avenue. It was after dark, and my partner mashed the button on the floor, holding it down until the siren peaked out. As this happened, the 6-volt electrical system maxed out, and all the vehicle's lights dimmed to less than 1 candlepower.

A few blocks down Lincoln Avenue, we arrived at the scene of a traffic collision. Two women were in one of the vehicles, which was wedged against a phone pole. The driver's door was caved in and wouldn't open, so I opened the back doors of our rig and started to fetch the Porto-Power tools (it would be another 10 years before the Jaws of Life were invented). While I was struggling to get the heavy case of tools out of the rig, my partner flexed those enormous biceps and opened the caved-in door with his bare hands. What a guy!

That old Ford rig of ours was both ugly and beautiful. Her styling was vertical and blunt, but her bright-red paint was without a blemish. Other stations had newer rigs but, to my mind, no one had more character than Rescue 11. Eventually, I passed probation and got to drive her.

I knew that Rescue 11 would be retired someday and sold at auction, and I intended to buy her when that happened, but raising a family and going to school diverted my attention. I assume she spent her final years as a plumber's truck in East Los Angeles and finally was crushed for scrap metal.

About two years ago, with family raised and school behind me, I began to look for a hobby car. Looking through *Hemming's Motor News*, I saw an ad for a '47 Ford half-ton panel truck. I traveled to Brainerd, Minn., to inspect the hulk of what was once a magazine delivery truck. A few weeks later, it was shipped to California.

The reincarnation of Rescue 11 is under way. At the present, she is completely disassembled, and the body is down to bare metal. Sometime next year, she will emerge in original color and markings. From the outside, she will look like the original item, but underneath and inside, she will have modern mechanicals.

Master builder Randy Clark is creating a new front subframe to accommodate independent suspension and disc brakes. Power will be supplied by a reworked 351-cubic-inch Ford Cleveland engine, running through a C-6 automatic transmission to a 9-inch differential. Creature comforts will include cruise control, a tilt steering wheel, air conditioning and a stereo.

Most important, it will be wired for a 12-volt electrical system.

In back, we hope to mount rescue equipment of the 1950s, including an oxyacetylene backpack torch, Stokes stretcher and MSA "demand-type air apparatus." If we can find one, we'll include an E&J Resuscitator-Inhalator-Aspirator, as well as a wood-and-canvas military stretcher, smoke ejector, and several coils of manilla rope (we had never heard of kernmantle in those days).

The main reason for replacing the original mechanicals with modern components is to make the "new" Rescue 11 comfortable and safe for long-distance travel. Meanwhile, if you've got a rescue rig that's special to you, be advised that it's less expensive to keep it around than to create a replacement 30 years later. But probably not as much fun.

Reincarnated

Back in 1992, I shared news of our efforts to create a replica of the first rescue rig I was assigned to-Los Angeles County Fire Department's "Rescue 11." When I last reported on it, she was a bare-metal hulk resting on jack stands.

The original Rescue 11 was a 1947 Ford half-ton panel truck, small and light-duty by today's standards. She was underpowered and overloaded with equipment that would now look primitive and cumbersome. I was a young kid, barely old enough to work for the fire department. Being trusted with responsibility for a rescue unit was awesome, and I loved it.

Slowly but surely, Randy Clark, my hot rodding partner, has created a masterpiece of automotive art. Rescue 11 has emerged with five gallons of red acrylic paint adorning her flawlessly straight body. The exterior is exactly like the original, complete with roof lights, diamond-plate rear step bumper and gold-leaf lettering. But she has received a heart transplant.

A 351-cubic-inch Ford Cleveland engine throbs beneath the hood. Its innards include a camshaft that makes the whole truck rock at idle. The C-6 transmission shifts gears with neck-snapping sureness. Creature comforts include air conditioning, leather seats with arm rests, electric windows and 100 amps of stereo power. (I know, it's not original, but I just couldn't resist.)

As an automotive restoration project, it sort of defies description. Rescue 11 isn't old enough to be a real antique. The modern running gear and interior rule it out as a restoration. It's not lowered, chopped or channeled, so it's not really a hot rod. But it attracts admiring glances, friendly waves, honks and thumbs-up gestures like nothing I've ever driven before.

In February, I decided to drive Rescue 11 to the Temecula Rod Run, an annual automotive event in Southern California. More than 1,200 cars were entered, including some truly beautiful rods and customs. I got there late and was assigned a parking place on a side street. As soon as I parked, a crowd formed. Nonstop for several hours, I answered questions about the truck, the whole function of rescue as an essential part of public safety, and Rescue Magazine.

Since an objective of the Rescue 11 project was to create a rolling icon for our magazines, the public reaction was gratifying. Driving home on Interstate 15, I was frequently boxed in by cars with drivers and passengers who wanted to get a closer look. We've since made covers for the roof lights and bought a magnetic "Not in Service" sign (just in case somebody along the way really needs to be rescued).

But the best was yet to come. About two weeks after the Temecula show, UPS delivered a plaque to my home. Of all the beautiful cars on display, Rescue 11 was judged to be in the Top 20. But the question remains: Is it an antique, a restoration or a hot rod? I guess it doesn't matter.

Thanks to some generous friends, we're beginning to restore vintage rescue equipment that will be mounted in the truck. We displayed Rescue 11 at the California Fire Instructor's Workshop in April in San Jose, Calif. We hope to take it to other shows where it can be enjoyed by rescuers and the public alike.

We're putting together a display board to be used at public events where the truck is displayed. We hope Rescue 11 will help educate the public about what you-as modern rescuers-are trained and equipped to do.

Recently, in the face of severe local government finances, we've heard suggestions that fire departments reduce their staffing or turn their functions over to private companies. But the fact remains that when the earth is quaking, the mud is sliding, the hazardous materials are spewing, the trenches are caving in, the bridges are collapsing, the rivers are rising or Amtrak is derailing, the public wants to be rescued promptly. They want enough rescuers to get the job done. They want their rescuers to be trained professionals-whether paid or unpaid-and they want them to be well equipped.

To convince the public of the importance of rescue, we need to get their attention. Rescue 11 is a tool to get the public's attention-and it seems to work. We hope to use it for conveying important information about what you do and how much you are needed.

But we can't do it alone. We urge you and your rescue team to develop your own method of attracting positive attention to the essential public safety function of rescue. Take your modern rigs and equipment to county fairs, school open houses, car shows and swap meets, and get close to your adoring fans. It's as much fun as it was 35 years ago.

The 70-Percent Margin

A couple of months ago, I wrote about the reservoir of goodwill I encountered while driving a restored 50-year-old fire-rescue truck across America. We logged nearly 8,000 miles and at least 20,000 smiles, waves, thumbs-up gestures and horn honks from other motorists.

The morning of Sept. 20th stands out in my memory. The previous day, I had presented a seminar for the North Central Texas Fire Chiefs Association in the Dallas area. Then, to avoid the heat and humidity, I decided to continue my journey at night.

The road from Dallas to El Paso is long and boring. After midnight, there's nothing on the radio, and the truckers even stop chattering on the CB. About 12 hours after leaving Dallas, the sun was coming up behind me, my mouth tasted awful, my eyes burned, my back ached and my stomach was sour. I'd been awake for 25 hours and Van Horn, Texas, was up ahead.

A Mercury Marquis with Michigan plates followed me off the Interstate. It tailed my shiny red truck to the Best Western motel. As I unwound my sore body and stepped out of the truck, the people in the Mercury - a man, his wife and their two preteen sons - approached me with smiles and a camera.

There has never been a time in my life when I felt less hospitable. But, just a day or two earlier, I'd read a survey report in USA Today about American institutions and trust. Rated at the top were fire departments, having earned the trust of more than 70 percent of Americans surveyed. Next highest were police departments (about 30 points lower).

Wow, what a great position to be in! It occurred to me that every one of us has an obligation to preserve that relationship of trust. That thought came back to me in Van Horn. More than anything, I wanted to be left alone. But I spent 10 minutes talking with the folks from Michigan, telling them about Rescue 11, and smiling for their camera. Then I rented a room and fell asleep.

A few days earlier, I had dropped in on a fire station in Conover, N.C. Those folks deserve a prize for the having the cleanest, best-maintained fire apparatus encountered on our '97 tour of America. In a few other places, we saw fire apparatus that looked and sounded worse than the local garbage trucks.

In a few places, in career, combination and volunteer departments, we saw fire stations that were filthy and unkempt. Several miles down the road, we found stations, including some older ones, kept as neat and spiffy as a Marine Corps barracks.

In most places, when we appeared unannounced at the door of a fire station, we were greeted promptly by people (both paid and unpaid) who were courteous and friendly. They seemed to realize that they are the temporary guardians of public facilities and that we're all responsible for that 70 percent margin of public trust. In a few places, we encountered sloppy, dirty, unshaven people who seemed perturbed that anybody would intrude on their private hideout (a publicly owned and financed fire station). "Yeah, whaddayawant?" was the greeting we got at one big-city station.

Some of America's firefighters work in some of America's worst neighborhoods. In those places, most cars look like refugees from a demolition derby. Most buildings are in a state of advanced deterioration. Trash is everywhere and so are the cockroaches. A duty shift in one of those neighborhoods can be full of calls to ugly places where foolish people have done stupid things to themselves and others.

So, do firefighters (the people Americans trust most) rise above it and set a higher standard? Do their engines and trucks, their stations and uniforms demonstrate pride, self-discipline, respect for property and a little elbow grease? Or, do they gradually let their vehicles, their buildings and their personal grooming and dress standards sink to the level of their neighborhoods?

In most locales, firefighters have accepted the higher standard, and they live by it. Unfortunately, however, in some places in America, fire stations and their crews resemble those found in third-world nations. Is it a matter of budgets? To some degree, but mostly it's a matter of pride. It doesn't cost much to clean and polish a fire engine, throw away junk that's accumulated on the apparatus floor, wash windows or paint grimy walls. What's the price of shaving before coming on duty, tucking in your shirttail and being courteous?

In Bethel, Ohio; Great Bend, Kan.; Earleigh Heights, Md.; Irving, Texas; Virginia Beach, Va.; and many other places we visited, the fire service is reflecting the pride that has earned the public's trust. In a few other places, the fire service has absorbed some of the ugliness and dysfunction of its immediate surroundings.

An old fire service tradition that deserves resuscitation is the Chief's inspection. Every month or so, a chief officer schedules a formal inspection of each station's quarters, apparatus, equipment and crew. A list of needed improvements is given to the company officer, with a reasonable period of time allowed for compliance. If corrections aren't made or underway when the Chief re-inspects, it is reflected in the company officer's performance evaluation.

The trust referred to in the *USA Today* survey didn't just happen. It's been earned by several generations of firefighters and their leaders. It is a wonderful affirmation of who we are and what we do. Take a look at your organization. Stand back and view it as an ordinary citizen might. Will your organization be remembered for building on that 70 percent margin of public trust or for squandering it?

Everything's Changed

I'm getting real tired of those folks who claim the fire service is stuck in the past. You've heard it ("200 years of tradition unimpeded by progress"), and so have I.

Sure, there are some fire service traditions that haven't changed much. Like being ready to do the job on a moment's notice. Like having an organization with some pretty clear lines of authority and responsibility. Or, like being the only outfit in town with the tools and the skills to cut thick metal, lift slabs of concrete, or deliver enormous quantities of water. What's wrong with that?

Earlier this summer, I parked my 50-year-old rescue truck (Rescue 11) next to a modern fire-rescue vehicle. We were at a fire service open house and the public was invited. While I was showing off the 80-pound E&J resuscitator that's mounted in my rig, a young guy from the modern rig next door pulled out a new 12-pound defibrillator. Talk about progress!

I opened up my Porto-Power box; it holds about 100 pounds of pre-1970s hydraulic spreading and cutting equipment, all of which was actuated by hand-pumped rams. The young fellow with the big rig promptly opened cabinets to display the most modern versions of spreading and cutting equipment-hydraulic and electric. Today, a crew can dissect a Dodge in the time it once took to offload and assemble the pieces of a Porto-Power.

When my rig was new, it was stationed with a Seagrave pumper. Rescue 11 had a little flathead V-8 under the hood and the Seagrave had a V-12. Neither of them had enough torque; kids on bicycles could beat us in a drag race. Responding to fires, the slightest hills forced us to downshift into first gear and crawl toward that growing pillar of smoke and flame in the distance. Have you mashed the pedal on a new Cummins or Detroit diesel? Now that's power.

During my first year in the fire service, I picked up a copy of one of the leading fire service magazines. The cover photo showed two fire chiefs in the foreground and billows of smoke in the background. They were facing each other, about 2 feet apart, and shouting at each other simultaneously. One was pointing an outstretched arm and finger to the east. The other was pointing to the west. That's the way they did it before incident command was devised. Talk about progress.

Forty years ago, a fire at a Catholic school in Chicago killed dozens of kids and their teachers. The building had open stairways, no sprinklers and no alarms. In the aftermath, building and fire codes throughout North America were upgraded and enforced. Today, a kid has a bigger chance of being shot at school than being trapped by a school fire.

I've spent much of this summer attending fire chiefs' conferences in the Southeastern, Northeastern and Midwestern states. To get a grip on just how much the fire service has changed, I've compared the chiefs I've met this summer with some of those I worked for in the early years of my career. Oh, the stories I could tell. It's enough to say that the new breed is a vast improvement.

From leather and canvas to Kevlar and Nomex, from street box alarms to mobile data terminals, changes have been phenomenal. From bad addresses and misdirected fire apparatus in the 1960s to enhanced 9-1-1 and GPS in the 1990s, very little is the same. Modern hose and nozzles bear little resemblance to the equipment used just two decades ago. Who says we haven't made any progress?

But the biggest change may be the hardest to measure-that is, public attitudes toward firefighters and the fire service. Not too many years ago, friends and neighbors of most career firefighters jumped at the chance to comment about days off and sleeping on duty at the firehouse. Friends and neighbors of many volunteer firefighters often made them the butt of bad jokes over fireground mistakes and pratfalls.

Starting about 1970, public attitudes began to change. Maybe folks started to realize that their local firefighters were often the first resource called to emergencies and the last to leave. When we started serving as medical first responders, our friends and neighbors may have noticed the sirens blowing throughout the night. Maybe they noticed and marveled at our powerful new apparatus and the modern tools and equipment we were starting to carry.

Maybe the new generation of fire chiefs impressed residents and business people as they got involved with local service clubs, charities and chambers of commerce. Maybe it was the favorable depictions of firefighters on television, in series like "Emergency!" and "Rescue 9-1-1."

Whatever the sources of the trust and admiration expressed by the public toward the fire service, it's something to be valued. Like anything of value, it can be lost. One way to squander it is to buy into a false image. To say that the fire service is stuck in the past ignores reality and chips away at a hard-earned asset.

7

Fire Chiefs

Simple Advice

You've got too many chiefs," I told the assembled fire department officials. I was speaking to the chief officers and management staff of a large fire department. As expected, several of them furrowed their brows and shifted in their seats as they heard me utter the unthinkable. Predictably, most of them glanced to see whether the top chief was reacting.

It was the end of a long study, including several weeklong site visits. I had become a familiar sight and a first-name acquaintance to many people at all ranks of the organization. I had dined with the troops, bunked in firehouses and responded on emergencies. I'd sat in on staff meetings, training sessions, performance evaluations and post-incident critiques.

"The number one problem of this department is routine communication upward and downward through the organization," I continued. The big chief, sitting up front, nodded slightly. Almost immediately, everybody else started to nod in agreement. It was true. It seemed almost impossible to promptly convey accurate and timely information in either direction.

"At least two of the five levels of chief officers in this department were established in hopes of improving communications,"

I said. The department is like many others that have made the same mistake. The assumption that another layer of authority between top and bottom will improve communication has been around for a long time, even though it almost always makes things worse.

None of this was a surprise to the chief of that department. I'd already given him a briefing. He knew what was coming, and he knew that the shock value of controversial statements by an outsider was important. His department was approaching the 21st century with a 1950s management culture. He couldn't change it without some help.

During that project, I saw and heard things that are common to most fire departments in the English-speaking world, both career and volunteer. Lack of trust is one example. Decades ago, the people at the top didn't trust the people at the bottom to do the right thing. So they created paper trails for everything, not to make sure that things got done, but to nail people when things went wrong.

Every chief in the department grew up with that system, and nobody had ever questioned it before. It was part of the organizational culture, and my message was attacking some of their most ingrained behaviors.

While working with that department, I frequently borrowed unoccupied desks to make phone calls or do my work. On those desks, I'd usually see copies of memos written by chiefs. In many cases, they'd been drafted in handwriting and given to a typist to clean up and finalize. Most of the memos were about really simple stuff, the kinds of things my secretary routinely takes care of without even telling me.

When asked how they learned what a chief officer was supposed to do, most said they simply did what they'd seen others do over the years. It became clear that the culture of the organization was still influenced by an old chief from the era of strong backs and weak minds. He had been mean-tempered, heavy-handed, abusive and intolerant of even honest mistakes.

A generation later, chiefs in that department still spend a lot of time covering their tracks as though the old man might rise from the grave.

Actually, the excessive levels of management, coupled with the fearful compulsion to get everything in writing and pass it through channels, has constipated the department's flow of information. But the worst effect has been at the company officer level.

With too many chief officers looking for important things to do, they've gradually robbed company officers of their authority. Unfortunately, most company officers have been too willing to forfeit it; they just rolled over. Their pay remains the same whether or not they're making the tough decisions.

The fire company is the basic unit of fire protection and EMS. The company officer is the only person who truly can control his people throughout the entirety of a duty period. To be effective, the company officer must have authority that matches the responsibility.

When chiefs oversupervise company officers, they erode that authority. Sadly, in many departments, nobody has ever seen what a fully empowered company officer can achieve. Instead, most company officers think of themselves as little more than firefighters with a fatter paycheck and bugles on their lapels. Their growth as leaders has been stunted because they've been taught to do less rather than challenged to do more.

The fire department I've described is typical; you may think it's your own. It's a product of generations of learned behaviors, many of which are no longer appropriate. It will not make a successful transition to the 21st century while embracing a culture from the 1950s. It must flatten its organizational structure, it must learn to trust its people, and it must drive decision making down to the lowest possible levels in the organization.

That's simple advice for a monumental task. It may take a generation or more to achieve, but it must be done.

Mike's Chief

"Good afternoon," I said into the phone. "I'm glad you're there Jim," said the voice on the other end. "I really need to talk to you." I recognized the voice immediately. We'll call him Mike for the duration of this column.

Mike started as a volunteer firefighter and decided to make the fire service his career. He has a good education, he's fit and well groomed, he writes and speaks well and he's genuinely likeable. After joining a career department in a city near his home, he advanced through the ranks quickly.

A couple of years ago, while I was traveling in his state, Mike invited me to join his family for a home-cooked meal. It was a memorable evening in a home filled with love and laughter. Later, he and I sat on his screened porch, smoked Dunhill Coronas and sipped Bushmills as twilight turned to night. Of course, we talked about the fire service.

He'd just been promoted to second in command. His boss, the new fire chief, had come from another city and was said to be progressive. After years of working under stagnant leadership, Mike was looking forward to a new era. "If he'll just lead the way," he said, referring to the new chief, "I'll work my heart out to make him successful."

Two years later, things were different. The new chief, it seemed, didn't live by his words. He often spoke of the need for open communications, but his staff learned quickly that the man had little patience for bad news. He urged his people to propose changes and improvements, but his reaction to those proposals usually depended on his prevailing mood.

"There are times when he's just downright abusive," Mike told me. "If something goes wrong, and he's in one of his moods, he'll berate an officer mercilessly-right in front of the rest of the staff. Every one of us is taking some kind of medication for stress, ulcers or high blood pressure."

"It's ironic," Mike said. "I often know when a problem in the department is developing and I know how to help the chief prevent it or solve it before it becomes a big deal. But he either shuts me out, wants complex information in two-sentence packages or throws a temper tantrum when he hears the bad news."

Mike was confused. On the one hand he was loyal to the chief, but unable to help him succeed; the boss had made open communication painful and expensive. On the other hand, Mike sometimes was tempted to unload on the man-to scold him when he was abusive. It was pretty certain his career would suffer if he ever did that.

When you and your family have deep roots in a community, you hate to even think about seeking a job elsewhere. But that's what Mike was considering when he called me. His wife is active in the community and has a part-time job she loves. The kids are thriving in school. "Is it fair to them for me to apply for a chief's job that would require us to move?" he asked.

The one element of his career plan that he couldn't control was luck or fate. To an extent, we can make our own luck. But there are times when the best of plans get derailed by things we have no control over. That's what happened to Mike-and to many of the rest of us at one time or another. The man he'd looked forward to working his heart out for had a moody, destructive side to his personality.

I couldn't advise Mike on what to do, but I helped him see the pros and cons of his options. He'll probably become the chief of another department in a year or two. His wife and children will move with him; they'll adjust and do well because they're strong, stable and supportive of one another (i.e., a family).

The saddest part of this story is Mike's chief. Is it possible he doesn't realize the damage caused by his unpredictable, abusive behavior? Doesn't he understand that he can succeed only through other people? Unless he's totally oblivious, he must know that you can't berate and humiliate people and then expect them to trust and respect you and work hard to make you successful.

So my question is whether a troubled man will recognize himself in this column. Sometimes the most abusive, insensitive people see themselves as just the opposite. Perhaps Mike's chief will read this and think, "How could any fire chief be so stupid as to act that way?" It's not a matter of intelligence; it's emotional stability that's needed. If you are Mike's chief, I hope you'll take this message to heart. Fess up to your shortcomings, apologize to the people you've hurt and seek some professional counseling. If you can learn to trust those around you and treat them with courtesy and respect all the time, they will make you a success.

If you can't, long after you're gone, the only thing people will remember about you is your worst behavior.

The Chief's Handicap

It's a good thing controversy sells magazines. Otherwise, this month's column might put us out of business. It all started when our editor Michelle Garrido sent me an e-mail: "You're next 'Burning Issues' column is due Monday." I drew a blank. It seemed I'd just turned in the last one; my creative well was dry.

Next morning, I was on my way to a meeting, driving northbound on I-15. As I passed the Lawrence Welk Resort and golf course near Escondido, Calif., I thought about my six iron. I wondered if it was still in the bottom of the lake. Intense emotion is a powerful generator of creative thought. That lake and that dastardly six iron brought back ugly memories of the day I quit golfing. Suddenly, my creative well refilled.

Some people, including my wife, insist that golf has therapeutic qualities. How can anything that makes you angry be good for you? Some guys have told me they clinch business deals while playing golf with potential customers. Who would want to do business with someone who shouts profanities at a little white ball?

Nearly every fire chief's conference I've ever attended had a golf tournament. Some guys look really cool, with expensive clothes, fancy bags, the latest clubs and a smooth swing that arcs with precision from way back here to way back there. But most of the guys look like their shoes don't fit, and they're trying to kill rattlesnakes with a baseball bat. They're usually called "hackers" or "duffers." I fit in that group.

Gossip among fire chiefs is pretty predictable. A chief with a golf handicap of 10 or less is usually the subject of admiration, envy and some jealousy (including suggestions that he cheats). Those who play as I did become the butt of jokes and ridicule when their colleagues get together. As a result, many chiefs either keep their handicap a secret, lie about it or humbly accept the demeaning labels. Before my six iron took the big swim, I was in the latter category.

For a long time, I felt self-conscious about my performance as a golfer. I thought it might help to join a country club. Now, my wife uses the country club, and I pay the monthly bill.

While I struggled with the game, took lessons and made a fool of myself, I also tried to function as the chief of a career fire department. That's when I heard the admonition that to maintain a handicap of 10 or less, golfers have to play 18 holes at least twice a week. To improve their game, they must play at least three times a week. Since then, I've presented this theory to a lot of good golfers, and they all agree.

At one point, I hired a golf pro to teach me how to play. In a moment of frustration, I asked him how many strokes it takes for a person to advance from beginning golfer to PGA pro. "About a million," he said. A million strokes divided by an average score of 85 equals 11,764 rounds (not counting driving range strokes). At four hours per round (47,058 hours), that's equivalent to 16 years (eight hours per day, seven days per week).

Since 1975, the job of a fire chief has become at least four times more difficult and complex. The list of new challenges includes EMS, hazmat, ethnic and gender diversity, vanishing volunteers, a revolution in personnel safety requirements (including fireground accountability systems), tax revolts, urban disorder and suburban school terrorism, "two-in/two-out" staffing, the Fair Labor Standards Act timekeeping, incident command systems and customer service.

I know I'm a lousy golfer, but I hope I was a better-than-average fire chief. I tried hard to keep my department on the leading edge of fire-service changes and challenges. Despite 50- to 60-hour workweeks, I could barely keep up with it all. My staff and I were forever working against deadlines, while putting out all the little personnel "brush fires" that ignite whenever a fire department is asked to change.

Which leads me to the point (and the controversy). Unless I could have reduced my workweek by 10 to 15 hours, there's no way I could have been a competent fire chief and a respectable golfer. Stated as a question, can fire chiefs with a golf handicap of 10 or less really do their job as well as it needs to be done?

I'd be first to admit that some people have a natural aptitude for golf-for example, those guys with the smooth swings, soaring drives, surgical chip shots and intuitive putts. Presumably, a few of them got that good with little effort, and they maintain their natural skills without practicing very often. If any of those people are working as fire chiefs they are probably wasting their talent and time. They should get a PGA card and make some real money.

Those of us without that natural talent for golf should stop hoping for miracles. It's never going to happen. Meanwhile, there are plenty of fire service challenges to occupy our time. It may not be as much fun as golf, but it's a lot more productive.

8

Getting Things Done Through People

Make-Believe Firefighters

Fighting fires is labor intensive and complex. That has been confirmed by the department of industrial engineering at a major university. The professors there studied a fire in a single-family dwelling and the response to that fire by a properly staffed, trained and equipped fire department. They were surprised by what they found.

"The attack and extinguishment of a fire in a single-family dwelling may represent the most complex, interdependent, time-sensitive set of tasks to be found in any working environment we've ever studied," the professors said (or words to that effect).

We can presume they've never studied the Patriot system that intercepts incoming missiles. Still, such a conclusion from a group of academic efficiency experts is pretty impressive.

"Complex" and "interdependent" means we've got to be able to depend on one another. Time-sensitive means things have to get done right away, or else. If that's the case, what do we do about make-believe firefighters? They're the ones who dress for the party but never make it inside.

Every fire department, career or volunteer, has one or more of them. While others crawl down a hallway, pushing a wall of flame into retreat, pulling a heavy, stiff hoseline from behind, make-believe firefighters open and close cabinets on the rig out in the street. "I just know those hall runners are in here someplace."

Sometimes, make-believe firefighters get promoted. One night, I rolled in on a fully involved triple-wide mobile home. You could see the fire from miles away. At the scene, two firefighters were wrestling with an interior hoseline. One of them fell through the floor. I helped pull him out of the hole, determined that he was OK and asked, "Where's your Captain?" "Haven't seen him since we got here," he said.

Outside, I found the Captain. He was clean and dry, and not wearing his SCBA. He was helping the next-door neighbors search for their frightened cat. What I said to that Captain is not fit to print. He was notorious for getting lost when the job got dirty or dangerous. Incidentally, he never hesitated to pick up his paycheck.

The first Fire Captain I worked for had seen combat action in the South Pacific as an infantry officer. He wouldn't hide from anything. But he also took pride in eating more smoke than compatibility with life would suggest. He participated in the selection of new firefighters for the department. They looked for people who would love to get wet and dirty, swear at a fire while knocking it down, and then go outside and vomit for the crowd.

Almost everything has changed since then, mostly for the better. But the concepts of risk, work and obligation have suffered grievously. Still, the real essence of fighting fires remains the same; it is hard physical teamwork that requires some calculated risks to meet our obligations to each other and to those we serve.

Which leads us to one person-the fire company officer. The company officer must get the job done with people who may have no prior background in dirty, risky work, and who've grown up in an era of ever-expanding "rights."

Meanwhile, thousands of new hazardous materials have been invented, some scary infectious diseases have come along, and terrorism has become more prevalent. Trying to keep firefighters and others out of harm's way, federal and state governments have given the first-line supervisor (fire company officer) a pile of safety regulations. Some firefighters interpret this as a "right" not to be injured.

In the face of such a daunting set of circumstances, some company officers will jump at a chance to search for the neighbor's cat, so to speak. But the good ones will seek and find the right balance between risks and results.

They'll recognize the need to create in their crew members a work ethic that mixes aggressive attack with intelligent strategy. That means the whole team working together on an interior attack or venting a roof, but also backing off when the incident commander opts for the defensive mode. If you're a real firefighter, you know there's nothing better than stopping a fire in its tracks, but there's nothing worse than losing one of our own to a derelict building that wasn't worth saving.

Company officers have lost a lot of power in recent years, and many of them have given it away. To chief officers who oversupervise. To personnel and safety bureaucracies. To unreasonable concerns about "the law." It's time to put the power back where it belongs-with the one person who has the greatest opportunity to influence and control those closest to the point of service: firefighters.

If a company officer finds that he or she has a firefighter who'd rather search for hall runners or hunt for the neighbor's cat than work a hoseline down a burning hallway, the process of training, motivation-and, if necessary, progressive discipline-should be started immediately. There is no place for make-believe firefighters.

Sex, Lies and the Workplace

Sex is such a wonderful thing. On the other hand, it can lure people into absolutely hopeless situations. For example, brainless escapades by a president who'll be remembered more for his zipper than for his leadership. Other examples include a Fire Battalion Chief who lost everything for a few moments of ecstasy and a pioneering firefighter who squandered her chance for a great career.

My former boss, Harvey Anderson, often said that natural instincts could not be contained if genders were mixed in a firehouse. I didn't accept that as a blanket statement. Sure, there would be some problems here and there but, all in all, if firefighters know the ground rules, they can be held responsible for their own behavior.

A few days ago, a retired fire buddy e-mailed me to restate his opinion that women don't belong in the fire service. He didn't offer a reason, but I remember one of his more entertaining firehouse tricks (igniting his own flatulence). Imagine the harassment suit over that!

I still disagree with him and with Harvey, but my confidence in firefighters of both genders has been shaken. It happened when a private ambulance guy told me of an event involving one of my Battalion Chiefs and our only female firefighter. The ambulance guy really enjoyed presenting me with a truly humiliating moment.

"One of your Chiefs and a female firefighter drove to my town in a Chief's car to pick up a fire department ambulance that had been painted at a local shop," the ambulance guy told me. "Before they left town, they found a remote parking lot and both of them crawled into the back of the ambulance."

I was stunned, wondering whether this was some kind of sick joke or dirty trick. "After about 20 minutes," the guy continued, "they got out of the ambulance, and the Chief was hitching up his pants. Then they drove away in two vehicles."

It was a Friday afternoon. Good thing, because I needed a couple of days to figure out how to handle the situation. Was it true? How could I be sure to get the truth? If it was true, what action should I take? Go public with the information, fire them both and set an example for others? Of course, that would also destroy their families and kill their careers.

In the end, I didn't involve lawyers or the human resources people. I chose to confront the two individually and demand the truth. I talked to the woman first. She admitted that the story was true and that she had not been coerced. Then I talked to the Chief. In the beginning, he tried to deny the story but broke down in a tearful admission when he learned that his paramour had come clean.

After a severe scolding, I told each of them that I had decided to spare their families from pain and embarrassment. I extracted promises of career-length, on-duty abstinence from both of them. They thanked me profusely. In exchange, I promised to go public with their secret if they ever again let their hormones overrule their brains while they were on duty.

A few weeks after I retired, a police cruiser spotted a fire department sedan in a secluded spot in the late-night hours. The windows were steamed. Inside, the policeman found the same two people breaking their promises to me. As soon as I heard about it, I kept my promise to go public. I hope they enjoyed their few minutes of steamy pleasure in the backseat of that red Chevy because it has cost them immensely.

This is not a tirade against sex. It really is a wonderful thing, even though most of the worst mistakes we make in life can be traced to that most powerful of human impulses. And, this is not an indictment of women in the fire service. I still believe that women bring a valuable dimension to our work and our organizations.

But any force as powerful as sex can devastate a working group if it's not contained and controlled at the work site. I'm worried about those who may assume that what's good enough for the White House Oval Office is good enough for the firehouse. In either place, the public's need for safety and security will be undermined by glandular compulsions.

Here are a few rules that may be helpful:

1. If you engage in on-duty sexual activity, you *will* get caught eventually.

2. Before you get caught, you *will* suffer lots of anxiety about your secrets and whether or not they'll be revealed.

3. Order *cannot* be maintained in a working environment where two or more workers have a sexual relationship.

4. The price you'll pay for illicit sexual conduct is *always* greater than the pleasure derived.

I really hate to burden you with all this dismal news and straight-laced advice. But if these words ever come to mind in a moment of brainless compulsion, and if they reverse the direction of your zipper, I will have done a good thing.

When Praise Backfires

The scene: *An appeal hearing regarding the discharge of Firefighter Smith. Smith's attorney is cross-examining Jones, the fire department officer who discharged Smith.*

Attorney: *"Did you recommend that Mr. Smith be discharged from his position as a firefighter with your department?"*

Jones: *"Yes, I did."*

Attorney: *"Why did you make that recommendation?"*

Jones: *"Because Mr. Smith was not meeting the minimum performance standards of our department."*

Attorney: *"But isn't it true that just 60 days before you fired Mr. Smith you completed a performance evaluation that praised him for improvements in his performance?"*

At some time or other, virtually every fire service officer will be faced with an employee or member whose performance needs improvement. Whether career or volunteer, most firefighters will on occasion have a supervisor who's dissatisfied with their performance. If the officer is a responsible professional (paid or unpaid), they won't make mountains of molehills or ignore real problems. An undeniable obligation of every fire service officer is to work constantly with members to meet or exceed reasonable standards of behavior and performance.

A basic principle of human behavior is that people are more responsive to praise than to criticism. If you criticize a worker's faults and weaknesses without acknowledging their strengths, you can't expect them to improve. Nothing inspires greatness in an individual more than praise for their virtues and achievements.

All learning is goal oriented. If an individual is told their performance must improve, they deserve to know specifically what's expected. In other words, their supervisor must give them some goals to shoot for. If changed behavior is one of those goals, the pathway to improvement will be long and difficult. Along the way, signs of progress must be acknowledged and further progress must be encouraged through positive reinforcement.

The public has a right to dependable, high-quality public health and safety services. That means every firefighter must meet or exceed reasonable standards of behavior or performance on a consistent basis, without prodding or hand holding by their supervisors.

The firefighter's direct supervisor must clearly identify areas of substandard behavior or performance; provide counseling on how to improve; work with the individual to develop a plan for improvement; and provide an atmosphere and opportunity for the individual to satisfy that plan, including plenty of positive reinforcement.

So what happens if the employee or department member ultimately fails? Despite some signs of progress along the way, what if their setbacks and shortcomings outweigh their improvements? What if the improvements seem temporary and fragile despite abundant praise and acknowledgement? After all, a fire department is a public safety agency, not an adult day care center. Firefighters must be responsible for themselves and each other.

After doing everything right, Jones decided that Smith would never be sufficiently stable or reliable to meet the department's standards. He recommended dismissal. Smith then requested a hearing and hired an attorney to represent him. Jones is now being cross-examined and the attorney is trying to demonstrate that the recommendation of dismissal is inconsistent with positive comments on Smith's interim performance evaluation just two months earlier.

If Smith's attorney does his job well, he will be an aggressive advocate for his client. He will question, challenge, dispute and test every bit of evidence that's being used against his client, including the testimony of Jones. But Jones has been well prepared by the fire department's attorney. This is apparent as he answers the question about positive comments on Smith's performance evaluation.

Jones: *"Yes, I did acknowledge some improvement on that report, but ... "*

Attorney: *"Thank you. You've answered the question."*

Jones: *"I'm sorry, sir, but that was only a partial answer. What I intended to say before you interrupted me was that the positive comments on Mr. Smith's interim performance evaluation should be seen as evidence of how hard we worked with him to help him succeed. It should not be seen as inconsistency. I'm sure you'll agree that nobody is inspired to improve if all they're getting is criticism. With Mr. Smith, I looked for any signs of improvement, no matter how slight or temporary, and I tried to use those signs to inspire him to keep working on his problems. I really wanted him to succeed, but in the end it became obvious that we couldn't depend on him to meet the department' standards. Because public health and safety are at stake, we had no choice but to let him go."*

An experienced trial lawyer probably wouldn't allow Jones to take control of the testimony this way, but it doesn't hurt to try. Even if Jones gets restricted to "yes" or "no" answers on cross-examination, his own lawyer can help him get this information into evidence during re-direct examination.

More important than trial tactics, however, is the fact that positive reinforcement remains the most powerful motivator of human behavior. Just because it might backfire at a future hearing or trial is no reason to not praise people when they do something right.

The Crummy Little Book

It's time for renewed efforts to support company officer development

A long time ago, on my first day as a fire company officer, I suddenly realized that I was not prepared for my new responsibilities. My department had given me an orientation, but it was all about filling out timecards, tracking overtime, ordering supplies and writing reports. They assumed I already knew how to give an order, which I didn't. Even worse, I didn't know what to do if I issued an order and somebody disobeyed it.

Five years later, I continued to learn through trial and error. Meanwhile, I met many other company officers also promoted to their position with little or no preparation. I decided to write about the experience and share with others some of my hard-earned lessons. For several months, at home and at Fire Station 7 in West Hollywood, I pecked away with two fingers on my Royal portable typewriter.

With about 300 pages of manuscript in hand, I looked for a publisher. I called my book Effective Company Command. I finally had to front the money to get it into print. I couldn't afford an editor so I published it with a lot of convoluted sentences and some embarrassing misspellings. Eventually however, thousands of copies sold.

Through the years, dozens of fire officers have told me that my book helped them get promoted and helped them in their jobs. If a crummy little book like Effective Company Command produces that kind of response, there must be a real need for quality preparation and guidance of company officers.

Captain Jeff Lytle works for one of America's fastest growing fire departments-the Henderson Fire Department near Las Vegas. Though we're a generation apart, his experience as a new company officer and his reaction to that experience have been very similar to mine. He has addressed the problem in a way that others could learn from. In the issue of FireRescue, he shared the details of his department's program of mentoring new or prospective company officers. (An Officer & a Regimen).

In November 2000, Captain Mike Ward and I presented a teleconference as part of the ICHIEFS Best Practices series. Mike's a veteran of the Fairfax County (Va.) Fire and Rescue Department and he writes a column on "Company Officer Development". Our teleconference topic was *Generation X, Y, Z: Managing Generations and Diversity.*

We approached the topic from the viewpoint that only one person can manage and resolve generational conflict and potential divisiveness in a diverse group of firefighters: the company officer. Judging by the response to the teleconference, there is growing recognition that this is the pressure point for both career and volunteer departments.

The career fire service may be the only remaining occupation in North America where people can enter as teenagers and where the vast majority remain with the same employer, in the same working environment, until they reach retirement age. Many volunteer departments have members who have remained active in one way or another for 40 years or more. This has many advantages. On the other hand, slow turnover allows an organization's culture to grow deep roots and successfully resist change.

Eventually, every fire chief learns that silent, invisible vetoes within the organization can derail their power to make things happen or change. Ultimately, every plan, program, memo or directive gets hashed out by the crews in the stations (without chiefs present). Only the company officer can control that environment.

For much of the past 25 years, doors of opportunity have been pried open for people who previously had been barred or discouraged from careers or membership in the fire service. In many firehouses, anger and dissension over affirmative action and consent decrees lurk just beneath the surface. Unless company officers are given the responsibility, training and authority to set the proper tone through personal leadership, those old wounds will continue to fester.

As a diverse group assembles in the confines of a typical firehouse, ethnic and cultural preferences and practices may clash. The company officer must maintain harmony and make certain that their team is capable at all times to meet the community's expectations-despite their differences. This calls for leadership of the highest order-the company officer who seeks to be popular above all else will surely fail.

The NFPA Fire Officer Standards and the IFSTA manual, *Fire Company Officer*, form important parts of the foundation. But they provide only minimum standards and really don't get the job done. For example, NFPA Fire Officer I Standard 2-2.1 states: "Identify methods used by supervisors to obtain cooperation within a group of subordinates and explain the supervisor's responsibilities in promoting cooperation within a group." Plenty of people can "identify methods" and "explain responsibilities" even though they may have no competence for leadership.

9

Ink Fights

The Imperfect Article

In July, *Esquire* magazine published an article about the deadly fire in Worcester ("The Perfect Fire"). With a couple of exceptions, it was well written and brought a human dimension to the cold statistics of the fire and its awful toll on the community.

By the time I got to the fourth page of the article, however, I was reminded of Norm Raymond. He'd been a firefighter for 20 years before I joined the department. Norm started his career somewhere back East and had lots of stories to tell. He told those stories with a gravelly voice honed by years of cigarette smoking, and he punctuated the stories with lots of profanity, especially the "f" word.

I was just a kid, still trying to figure out how to act in adult company. Norm was a popular man. The other guys seemed to respect him. They always laughed at his jokes. Of course, I wanted to be respected and popular too. So I started using profanity in the fire station, including the "f" word.

It seemed strange to hear myself saying that word. It had never been used in my home. Once, while watching my father fix something in the garage, I heard him say it when he hit his finger with a hammer. So, when I started to punctuate my firehouse conversation with profanity, it was unnatural and out of character. It didn't seem to make me any more popular either. No matter how many "f" words I threw into a conversation, Norm and the other guys still treated me like the dumb new kid.

In those days, when we had a visitor in the station, everyone-including Norm-cleaned up his act. Even if it were a deliveryman looking for directions, the profanity would stop while he was there. A couple of times, a newspaper reporter spent some time with us while preparing stories about the life of firefighters. Almost instinctively, the profanity disappeared from the firehouse banter. After all, our public image was at stake.

Somewhere during that phase of my life, I made a conscious decision to clean up my mouth. It wasn't a religious thing. I'm not a prude and I enjoy funny jokes-even if they're off-color. I still let loose with a four-letter word now and then. It occurred to me that the habitual use of profanity is nothing more than a crutch for undeveloped or impaired language skills. Why would anybody want to draw attention to that disability?

Meanwhile, numerous social influences have degraded our language. Have you been to an R-rated movie lately? Have you listened to any rap music? Have you watched an HBO comedy special? Have you listened to the skateboarding 12-year-olds in your neighborhood? The infamous "f" word is close to becoming the most frequently uttered word in the American vocabulary.

That's what struck me as I read the *Esquire* article. Did Sean Flynn, the writer, pepper it with "f" words just to add color, or is that the way the guys at Worcester were talking when the writer visited them? If that's the way the guys were talking, why? I hope that's not the way they talk at home in front of their parents, wives and children.

The *Esquire* article made me feel that I knew the six brave men who had lost their lives in that worthless building. Their personal and family backgrounds revealed most of the emotional, social and financial ups-and-downs that all of us have faced. Unfortunately, the well-written story of their lives and their ultimate sacrifice was marred by tasteless profanity that added nothing to the story.

Someday, the grandchildren of those deceased firefighters will look through the scrapbooks and other mementos of the day their grandfathers died. One of the mementos will be a copy of the Esquire article and it will still contain the trashy language.

By that time, the "f" word may be as acceptable as "darn" or "heck." Maybe those grandchildren won't even notice the profanity. On the other hand, maybe the pendulum will have swung in the other direction between now and then. Social trends seem to swing from one extreme to another. If our society begins to recognize profane words as only crutches for the verbally impaired, maybe a future generation will bring decent language and proper English into fashion.

No matter what happens in the future, clean language will never go out of style, and the superb reputation of firefighters will never be enhanced by public use of profanity. No matter where it's published, good writing does not get better when "f" words are used as a substitute for exclamation marks. The Worcester firefighters deserved a magazine article that was at least as dignified as their funeral.

Wall Street Junk Journalism

The *Wall Street Journal* enjoys a reputation for accurate reporting on matters of business and finance. On occasion, they stray into other topics with mixed results. Example: On February 7, the Journal published an article by staff reporter Robert Johnson about the American fire service, "As Blazes Get Fewer, Firefighters Take On Some Eclectic New Roles."

Johnson opened with the fact that the number of structure fires in the United States has decreased 40% in recent years. Meanwhile, he reported, the ranks of paid firefighters have increased by 20%. If that statement is accurate, the fire service has created 45,000 new firefighter jobs. To a typical businessman reading the *Wall Street Journal*, this would appear a classic example of featherbedding-employing extra workers with little or nothing to do. But that assumption by Johnson and his readers would miss the most significant point.

In 1970, the vast majority of small towns in the United States received fire protection from volunteer fire departments. In the interim, social and economic factors have increased the population of many small towns and changed the lives of most people who live in them. Especially during daytime hours, it is increasingly difficult for volunteer fire departments to muster a crew to fight a fire or extricate a crash victim. Thus, almost every town or city with a population of more than 9,000 has hired firefighters to supplement the volunteers.

Johnson made no mention of this phenomenon. Instead, he left readers with the impression that more people were hired to do less work. What's more, a typical business person reading the *Wall Street Journal* would naturally relate that impression to their familiar business environment. Without more information or a proper frame of reference, their reaction surely would be negative.

In 1970, the U.S. population was 203 million. The ratio of paid firefighters to citizens was 1.13 per 1,000. In February 2001, the U.S. population reached an estimated 278 million. Even with the additional 45,000 positions, the ratio of paid firefighters to citizens was .99 per 1,000. Mr. Johnson never mentioned this fact in his article.

The article's headline proclaimed firefighters have taken on some "eclectic new roles as blazes get fewer." The Kansas City Fire Department, he noted, answers about four times as many alarms today as it did in the mid-1970s-mostly auto accidents, heart attacks and kittens stuck in trees, the article states-but the number of fires has held steady at around 1,200 a year. Unmentioned was the fact that real people, many of them taxpayers, created the four-fold increase in demand for emergency services.

The *Journal* article's questionable research was most glaring when the author made reference to unnamed "government finance analysts." Reportedly, these bean-counters claim "nonfire medical emergencies, such as traffic accidents, could be handled more efficiently by a team of two paramedics arriving on the scene in an ambulance, rather than a crew of three or four helmeted firefighters clad in heavy protective suits aboard a gas-guzzling firetruck."

Obviously, Mr. Johnson and his unnamed efficiency experts have never seen a car crash with trapped victims and spilled fuel. Obviously, they don't know that the helmets and heavy garments protect against broken glass, razor-sharp metal, exploding air bags, battery acid and flammable fuel. The "more efficient" team of two paramedics would need to wear the same gear in order to protect themselves and comply with governmental safety requirements. Further, they would need a much larger vehicle resembling a "gas-guzzling firetruck" to carry all the necessary extrication equipment: hydraulic spreaders and cutters, winches and wedges, chains and cribbing.

No matter how well trained and equipped, it would prove impossible for a crew of two paramedics to simultaneously extricate and treat trapped and injured auto crash victims. But a typical business person reading the *Wall Street Journal* would not know that.

Apparently for dramatic effect, Mr. Johnson included another quote by the unnamed number-crunchers: "On many such calls, the only equipment used on a new $500,000 firetruck might be heart-reviving defibrillators or other paramedic gear." Nobody mentioned that, just as likely, the fire apparatus could be a 20-year-old rig with 150,000 hard miles on its odometer.

What's worse, Johnson ignored the motto of respected management expert Peter Drucker: "form follows function." America's most respected business publication focused on *form* (the size and price of the vehicle) rather than *function* (providing mobility and tools for a group of employees who can perform multiple tasks). By concentrating on the size and price of the vehicle, the *Journal* article missed an important principle of successful businesses-achieving greater productivity by using the same employees for several jobs.

Either Robert Johnson is a lazy journalist or his editor hacked his work. A few years ago, *Washington Post* reporter Janet Cooke lost her job and Pulitzer Prize for inventing a little boy she featured in a heart-wrenching series of articles. If Robert Johnson's "government finance analysts" really exist, why didn't he name them? If Johnson invented them and their opinions, is he any better than Janet Cooke?

It's Public Safety, Stupid!

Last month's "Burning Issues" focused on an article published in the Feb. 7 *Wall Street Journal* : "As Blazes Get Fewer, Firefighters Take On Some Eclectic New Roles." Written by Journal staff reporter Robert Johnson, the article purported to analyze the American fire service in advance of the expected adoption of NFPA Standards 1710 and 1720.

In my last column, I felt obliged to criticize the *Journal* for publishing poorly researched conclusions, based in part on the purported statements of unidentified "government finance analysts."

One of Johnson's most glaring omissions: the ratio of paid (career) firefighters to population. He pointed to a 20% increase in the number of paid firefighters, but failed to relate that to coincidental increases in population. He also failed to mention that there are fewer volunteers, requiring small towns in every state to employ a core staff of paid firefighters. I pointed out that, according to my research (the U.S. Census Web site, www.census.gov, and the *World Almanac and Book of Facts*), the United States had 1.13 paid firefighters per every 1,000 citizens in 1970. Early this year, that ratio dropped to .99 per 1,000. If, as Johnson reported, passage of NFPA Standards 1710 and 1720 prompt fire departments to hire 30,000 more "firemen" nationwide, the ratio would change to 1.07 per 1,000-still less than 31 years ago.

This month, I'd like to address the thread of distorted logic that ran through Johnson's report: If there are fewer fires, fire department budgets and staffing should be cut. After all, when sales of Gateway computers or Chrysler cars drop, workers get laid off. Why shouldn't fire departments expand and contract as demand for services rise and fall?

Because it's public safety, stupid! As administrators of public safety, fire personnel must handle fires, auto crashes, building collapses, floods, earthquakes and medical emergencies. These events remain-as always-unscheduled and unpredictable.

These calamities are time-sensitive, life-threatening and labor-intensive. You never know when they'll occur, but when they do, we need lots of trained and equipped people very quickly.

If the number of fires has declined by one-third, should we close every fire department for eight hours of every 24? Or should we reduce four-person neighborhood fire companies to 2.66 firefighters to cut costs? Neither option ensures prompt, reliable public-safety services. In a civilized nation, that's what the public expects-and they have a right to it. The public understands the difference between business and public safety. Business is about taking risks in pursuit of profit. Public safety is about preventing, minimizing and controlling risks.

Still, the *Journal* article never noted that the American fire service has adopted some smart business practices to give taxpayers more for their money. Specifically, most firefighters receive cross-training to provide emergency medical and rescue services in addition to fire protection. A few days after the *Wall Street Journal* article appeared, I boarded a plane operated by America's most profitable airline. The flight attendants were cross-trained as ticket agents. At the end of each flight, those same flight attendants clean the cabin in preparation for the next flight. Their boss has received much praise for maintaining a workforce that's willing to do more than one job for a reasonable wage.

If we can believe the *Wall Street Journal*, this flexibility "irks many local administrators, who think fire department budgets need to be cut." It's too bad the article failed to name any of those local administrators because we'd like to rub their noses in the economic and statistical facts I've mentioned. Short of that opportunity, we wonder why the Wall Street Journal couldn't see the good business sense of using firefighters for multiple public-safety roles.

Again relying on unnamed sources, Johnson claimed that "some consultants who study municipal services say fire departments' emergency medical aid comes at a premium cost." He then reported that privately employed paramedics typically make only 75% of the wages and benefits of firefighters. That's true-and that's the reason most private paramedics live at or below the poverty level. That's the reason there's so much turnover among private paramedics. *Example:* Several years ago in one major Midwestern city, the city auditor found that more than half their private paramedics had been on the job for less than one year.

The nation's best-known financial publication completely missed an important economic fact: Paid firefighters remain ready for public service, like a standing army. Even though Johnson's anonymous sources may not like it, the cost of that standing army is a given. The infrequent but unpredictable occurrence of fires results in surplus production capacity.

When firefighters accept responsibility for rescue and emergency medical services, the costs for those additional duties prove marginal (over and above the preexisting fixed costs). In many locales, fire departments generate ambulance revenues that equal or exceed those marginal costs. Any public administrator who gets irked by this businesslike approach to public-safety services clearly operates outside their level of competence.

The Cost of Living

For the third consecutive month, I'm responding to an article published in the Feb. 7 *Wall Street Journal* ("As Blazes Get Fewer, Firefighters Take On Some Eclectic New Roles"). Written by *Journal* staff reporter Robert Johnson, the article purported to analyze the American fire service in advance of the official vote on NFPA Standards 1710 and 1720.

I've read the *Journal* for years, and I've generally trusted its reporting on financial matters. That's why Johnson's distorted logic and the unfounded conclusions attributed to unidentified "government finance analysts" distressed me. If those "analysts" really exist, Johnson should have identified them before they could cause any further harm to public health and safety.

According to Johnson's anonymous sources, private ambulances often arrive on emergency scenes more quickly than fire trucks. He cited a recent four-month study in Kansas City showing that city firefighters arrived on scene in four minutes or less on between 60 and 70% of EMS calls. He failed to mention that the contractual response-time standard for ambulances in Kansas City is nine minutes on 90% of calls. Even if the ambulances met that standard, did Johnson's sources suggest that a five-minute difference in response times proves insignificant for cardiac arrest and penetrating-trauma victims?

The flawed article again stumbled into the trap of form-versus-function when Johnson reported that "one hook-and-ladder truck costs more than a half dozen ambulances." If his sources had given him the straight scoop, they would have informed him that departments spread the cost of a ladder truck over its life (20 years or more). Likewise, they spread the cost of six ambulances over their useful life (about five years). After four replacement cycles of the ambulances, the total net cost would equal twice that of the ladder truck. These are basic business principles. How could the esteemed *Journal* not see these economic facts?

On a similar note, when Johnson made the ladder-truck-versus-ambulance comparison, he seemed to suggest that a community would find it cheaper to operate six ambulances rather than one ladder truck. If his sources hadn't bamboozled him, Johnson would have recognized that labor costs-not the price of vehicles-remain the principal economic factor in any enterprise-government or business.

"Over the years," Johnson reported, "firefighters have been designated as the emergency 'first responders' in about 60% of U.S. communities, a niche that many fire departments have carved out for themselves as the incidence of fires has declined." Actually, in 94% of the nation's 200 most populous cities, the local fire department provides medical first-response services, but they didn't carve out that role for themselves.

As early as the 1920s, some fire departments reacted to the need for prompt, on-scene first aid for victims of sudden illness or injury. In my first year as a firefighter (1957) two-thirds of the calls we responded to were medical in nature. About 30 years ago-after the invention of CPR but *before* the decline in the incidence of fires-some highly esteemed physicians and public health authorities concluded that too many people died of cardiac arrest while waiting for an ambulance. Medical journals cited quick response by trained firefighters as the solution.

This evolution of lifesaving was born of necessity and encouraged by physicians. Inspired by medical research and the recommendations of national health organizations, 93% of fire department first-response units now carry automated defibrillators. The *Journal's* assertion that firefighters have created medical first response as some kind of self-protective niche is downright wrong and defamatory. It misrepresented an important chapter in the history of public health and safety.

Johnson failed to mention that American firefighters are also the responders of last resort. The local fire department is the only local government agency that can't turf an emergency to a higher level agency. If a fire won't go out, or an overturned rail car won't stop leaking chlorine, fire departments can't call the state police or the feds to take over. If something gets too hot, too stinky, too gooey or too messy, eventually the fire department will respond to cool it down, put it out or clean it up.

Every inch of space in a publication is valuable and should inform, educate or entertain. A lot of space was wasted in the Feb. 7 *Journal.* We think the editors should redeem themselves with an accurate, well-researched article about the increased hazards of building fires. In large part, the *Journal* has fostered Wall Street's fixation on short-term profits above all else. The resultant attitude has produced cheaper, lightweight construction innovations and dangerous storage practices that kill firefighters.

Johnson and his anonymous sources should confront the issue of defensive vs. offensive firefighting operations. If those financial analysts dislike the prospect of hiring enough firefighters to do the job safely, will they tell residents and business people that they and their property are expendable? Of course, not. That's why they chose to remain anonymous.

10

Keep the Lawyers Out of This

From Dumb to Dumber

One of America's major fire departments has lost several multi-million dollar lawsuits over its dispatching on medical emergencies. The problem started years ago when the city actively encouraged citizens to dial 9-1-1 for police, fire and medical emergencies, without conditions or exceptions. Nationwide, 9-1-1 has become the universal symbol for help.

The city in question bought one set of protocols (flip cards). It then modified the cards and attempted to train its dispatchers about how to use them for calls requesting medical assistance. If used *properly*, the protocols would guide the interrogation process so the dispatcher could send emergency resources based on medical condition and need. Also, the protocols could guide dispatchers in providing post-dispatch (prearrival) instructions to callers while emergency units responded.

The fire department in the opening example has provided emergency ambulance service for many years. For most of those years, the city's leaders treated that service as a stepchild, responding to its need for more resources only when a publicized crisis occurred. Thus, as the public caught on to 9-1-1, demand for ambulance service increased much faster than the number of ambulances. So, the dispatchers became the pressure point. They started deciding who would get an ambulance and who wouldn't. For those who didn't qualify, the dispatchers offered a phone number for private ambulances.

Denying emergency ambulance service is always risky, but the risk can be managed by using time-tested protocols, thoughtful dispatcher training, good supervision, ongoing training and a quality management program. In the city we're talking about, the dispatchers received the flip cards but not much else. Before long, some of the dispatchers began freelancing, trying to apply the protocols from memory, if at all. If asked, most couldn't locate the training manual issued to them when hired.

Because the number of ambulances didn't keep up with population growth and demand, the dispatchers were instructed to ration them to only those cases that involved "life-or-death emergencies." Their unskilled managers and supervisors criticized and disciplined quickly but rarely dispensed any positive feedback for jobs well done. Meanwhile, a culture of discourtesy, disrespect and impatience evolved in the dispatch center. It became an angry place and the unhappiness began to affect how employees treated callers.

The protocol (flip) cards all bear the boldly printed words, "When in doubt-send." In several cases over a period of years, where the facts about the caller's information should have raised doubts, dispatchers deviated from the protocols and denied ambulance service to dying people. When that happened, the dead person's survivors usually got mad. The most effective tool they had was a lawsuit. After a few of those lawsuits cost the city some really big bucks, the people in charge went from dumb to dumber. They looked to the city's lawyers for advice on how to dispatch.

Prompted by the lawyers, the fire department now sends too many resources on most calls. These days, it's not uncommon to have a street filled with fire apparatus, ambulances and staff cars for a relatively minor medical emergency. The firefighters know this over-reaction makes no sense to anybody but the city's lawyers.

The whole concept of prioritized emergency medical dispatching (EMD) was carefully designed to provide the appropriate response-without undue denials of service and without unnecessarily tying up too many resources. If prioritized EMD has a fault, it is the assumption that all public officials would be smart enough to implement and operate the system as it's supposed to operate.

In many places, the people in charge are smart enough to make prioritized EMD work and keep it working the way it should. Their success makes it easy to criticize those other places. Sadly, in too many of those other places, the dispatch center is controlled by people who seem to have been promoted or elected beyond their levels of competence. When incompetent leaders allow the system to go haywire, people get hurt and lawsuits occur.

When the lawsuits create a crisis, the leaders-oftentimes at the suggestion of their lawyers-overreact. Why must we make it so difficult? The public has been offered a service they can access by merely dialing three digits (9-1-1). They accept that offer more than anybody expected. So, there are two possible solutions: 1) revoke the offer; or 2) manage the demand for service intelligently. There's no politician foolhardy enough to revoke the offer, so that leaves only one option.

The key word: *intelligently*. Dispatch centers cannot be a dumping ground for hand-me-down managers and supervisors. Dispatchers cannot be treated as disposable employees. The concept of prioritized EMD cannot be treated as optional procedures.

If dispatch errors cause big-buck lawsuits, employ a simple solution. Utilize a current, nationally standardized emergency medical dispatch program, learn how to do it right, treat dispatchers as professionals and train them accordingly, select and train good supervisors, and implement a continuous quality management program. If those simple tasks are more than your organization can master, keep the checkbook handy. You'll need it.

Unfinished Business

At least a hundred cops have told me they'd rather face an armed crook than enter a burning building. Like most of you, I'd fight a thousand fires to avoid wrestling with one hallucinating dope fiend.

Cops get lots of training to prepare them for hostile, irrational and dangerous people. Police recruits study illustrated textbooks showing the proper restraint methods, including some extreme examples for situations where all else fails. From handcuffs and batons to tear gas and firearms, cops have the equipment to deal with people who threaten themselves or others. That's their job, and despite lots of second-guessing from critics who've never been there, our colleagues in law enforcement usually get the job done with little or no permanent damage.

Until about 20 years ago, firefighters didn't worry much about handling unruly, disruptive people. But the expansion of the fire service's role into EMS coincided with growing public abuse of mind-altering drugs and the widespread release of psychiatric patients from institutions to the streets.

Five times in recent years, I've been asked to defend firefighters who allegedly used excessive force or improper techniques to restrain patients. In every case, the patient was either wildly abusive, combative, irrational, inhumanly powerful, incoherent-or all of the above. In every case, the firefighters could not revert to their training or their textbooks for a simple reason: EMT and paramedic training programs ignore the topic and textbooks dance around it.

One firefighter/paramedic had faced an irrational patient who reached in his gun cabinet for a weapon. They ended up wrestling. There were no police officers on scene. The firefighter subdued the man with a closed-fist jab to his face, which broke his cheekbone. A jury decided the firefighter used reasonable force under the circumstances.

After firefighter/paramedics placed an unruly, drunken female on a gurney and applied soft restraints to her arms and legs, she continued to raise her head, curse and spit at the rescuers. One of the medics forced her head down onto the gurney, pressing on her forehead with the heel of his hand, his fingers laced through her hair. One of the woman's drinking buddies later alleged that the paramedic had violently pulled her hair. An investigator for the State Health Department believed the woman's drinking buddy and disbelieved the paramedic, who almost lost his license as a result.

Paramedics were called to a casino where security officers had detained a drunken, unruly man. The medics were asked to check the blood sugar of the detainee, who was straining at his handcuffs and making contorted facial gestures and animal-like sounds. The medics complied with the request, also checked lung sounds and assessed for distended neck veins, sweating, shortness of breath, and nausea, all of which were negative. They kept enough distance to prevent the man from biting them and left him with security personnel. Next day, the man had a heart attack and the paramedics were accused of being negligent.

These descriptions don't fully describe the events or the outcomes, but they spotlight another challenge for which the fire service is unprepared. EMS training programs and textbooks give scant attention to patients with a violent mental short circuit. Textbook editors, publishers and curriculum writers know the real truth about how to control violent, disruptive and unruly patients would be controversial. They dispose of the topic with a few generalities and bland safety warnings.

The only descriptive article for fire/ EMS personnel on restraining violent patients was published in September 1980 ("Rules of Restraint," *JEMS*). Among other techniques, the article recommended grabbing the patient's hair to keep them from injuring themselves or others. A photo of the technique included in the article looked barbaric-to people who've never had to control a paranoid schizophrenic or a hallucinating body builder.

To my knowledge, no fire department has trained its people what to do and how to do it when faced with these dangerous situations. To my knowledge, no fire department has amended its operations manual to include clear-cut directions on what to do or not to do when violent patients try to hit, bite, scratch, spit at, or otherwise injure first responders or firefighter/medics.

Should firefighters be disciplined if we don't like the way they handle violent patients? It's like telling firefighters to enter a burning building, but failing to provide them with necessary equipment or training-then punishing them when we don't like the way they perform.

For the most part, law-enforcement agencies are unhappy places to work. Every day and night, street cops face situations for which they are damned if they do and damned if they don't. As often as not, their bosses are afraid to back them up.

We've got a similar situation developing in the fire service. The solutions may not be pretty or politically correct. But the alternative is to ignore the problem and throw a few firefighters to the wolves when the ugly reality of the street conflicts with a sanitized view of how things should work. The experts who write the textbooks, training manuals and regulations have some unfinished business.

11

Bureaucratic Foibles

Dog Years & the Chain of Command

The North American fire service is undergoing a massive transition. In both career and combination departments, yesterday's leaders have begun to retire. For the most part, smart, well-educated and dedicated people will replace them. Still, issues will pop up for which the new leaders will find themselves unprepared. One of those concerns is the chain of command.

Traditionally, fire department leaders developed their leadership styles by mimicking those they had served under. Therefore, if the previous generation's fire chiefs were reluctant to trust their subordinates-failing to give them authority commensurate with responsibility-the next generation was likely to make the same mistake.

The words, authority and responsibility, when used in conjunction with one another, raise one of the most critical issues in any organization-but particularly in a fire department. That is: Authority must always be commensurate with responsibility. To give an individual the responsibility to achieve a goal or accomplish a task, but fail to give that person the necessary authority to follow through creates a recipe for failure.

In emergency situations there can be no argument.

Operating within the chain of command remains essential for effective action and risk reduction on the fireground. That's not the problem. The problem is rigid enforcement of the chain of command in routine, nonemergency actions and decisions.

Consider the example of a fire department with an ambulance service. The department's EMS billing and collection process and its EMS quality improvement and research projects require detailed and complete documentation of each medical event and patient treated and/or transported. Often, the EMS administrative staff members are in nonsworn (civilian) positions. To strictly enforce the chain of command, all formal communications between these staff members and paramedics would have to go through the EMS program manager (a chief officer), then to the district chief of the affected platoon, then to the paramedic's company officer, then to the paramedic.

Let's say the EMS quality manager needs more information on several patient transports. Should this staff person be required to request the additional information through the EMS office manager, then the EMS program manager, then the respective ambulance crews' district chiefs and then their company officers? This kind of rigidity would paralyze the organization. A more appropriate action would provide a blanket authorization for the quality manager to make direct contact with paramedics and/or their direct supervisors (company officers) except for extraordinary situations.

What if a fire pumper loses a fan belt on a Saturday night? Rigidly enforced, the chain of command would require the company officer to notify the battalion chief, who would then contact the assistant chief of the operations bureau, who would then contact the assistant chief of the services bureau, who would then contact the head mechanic, who would then assign a mechanic to make the repair.

Again, this rigid application of the chain of command would paralyze the organization. Days could pass before all the notifications could be made and permission granted. Meanwhile, a pumper would stay out of service with a relatively minor problem.

Some of the most striking differences in fire departments in North America arise from the varying degrees of delegated authority. Stated differently, it's often a matter of how much trust the leaders of the organization have in their subordinates. Generally speaking, the most progressive organizations have entrusted their people to communicate across and around the formal lines of authority in routine (nonemergency) matters.

That would include a company officer or battalion chief making direct contact with the duty mechanic without having to go through channels. It would allow a civilian staff member such as an EMS quality manager to make direct contact with paramedics, on an as-needed basis, without asking for permission through proper channels to do so.

In many line-and-staff organizations, strict conformity to the chain of command in all requests and communications has proven merely an effort to cover everybody's butt. If everyone in the chain of command is notified or asked for permission about everything that happens, nobody will ever be uninformed and everybody in the chain of command can pass judgment on administrative issues or questions.

However, the comfort and security of never being surprised or uninformed bears a big price. A fire department that requires strict conformity to its chain of command might be described, for lack of a better term, as constipated. Not only will progress at all levels slow to a snail's pace, but decision-making inevitably will be drawn to ever-higher levels within the organization. Before long, everyone below the top position (such as the fire chief) will lose the instinct to act decisively. Ultimately, the fear or unwillingness to make decisions or take decisive action without approval in advance will cripple even emergency operations.

In a line-and-staff organization, we can find the keys to avoiding excess rigidity in the following organizational beliefs, behaviors and attitudes, which most have difficulty achieving and sustaining:

Trust: The organization's leadership must have the ability and willingness to delegate routine decisions and actions to subordinates without the requirement of prior notification. As much as anything, confident leaders produce trust.

Restraint: The organization's leadership must have the ability and willingness to accept the fact that some decisions made and actions taken by subordinates may not meet their expectations or whims, and the self-discipline to resist intervening unless absolutely necessary. In the latter situation, a critical or negative reaction by the organization's leaders will blunt or nullify the delegation of routine decisions and actions.

Common Sense & Good Judgment: Those who accept delegated authority must exercise it responsibly. They must recognize their authority is extremely valuable, but extremely fragile. If they abuse it by failing to use common sense and good judgment, they will lose it.

Rigid, dogmatic compliance with the chain of command in routine matters may have worked well for the fire service in the 1800s. But we now live in a time when everything happens in dog years (seven times faster than human years) or faster. As early as 1911, a requirement that every manager sign off on routine decisions was considered bad form. In that year, Frederick W. Taylor described the exception principle of good management: A manager is required to get involved only in exceptional cases. In Taylor's words, "the exception principle frees the manager to take care of other and more important responsibilities."

No fire department can function effectively if it's focused on getting permission to perform routine tasks from everybody in the organizational chart. Let's hope the new generation of fire service leaders is intelligent and confident enough to trust their people, to delegate authority, and to free themselves to take care of those other and more important responsibilities.

Rat Calculus and Ugly Children

When the so-called founding fathers designed the structure of government for the United States of America, they defined three branches: executive, legislative and judicial. I'm sure it seemed reasonable at the time, before the discovery of electricity and petroleum. They couldn't have imagined that the government they had created would evolve to produce a fourth branch.

Over time, with the growth and complexity of all levels of government, the bureaucratic branch has emerged. In many ways, it exercises more power and independence than the other three. Theoretically, the bureaucracy is under the control of the executive branch, but any appearance of executive branch control over the bureaucracy is symbolic and temporary.

My opinions on this topic may seem cynical, but they're based in large part on a lifetime of working in and around government bureaucracies. For years, I've seen and heard career bureaucrats play a game of apparent deference, obedience and cooperation while quietly implementing their own agendas in tiny steps that go unnoticed for the most part.

In Washington, I've seen and heard career bureaucrats react to a "congressional request." (That's a letter from a member of

Congress to a federal agency inquiring about a program or an action taken by the bureaucracy.) Bureaucrats spend days fashioning a response that will sidestep the question, confuse the matter beyond all comprehension or dredge up arcane regulations to justify action or inaction.

It's a game, and the bureaucrats always win, even if they have to testify at a congressional hearing or wait for a new administration. The head of the executive branch (the president) nominates cabinet secretaries and administrators of federal agencies (the bureaucracies). The senate (in the legislative branch) reviews and confirms most of those appointees. Usually, there's a lot of hoopla about how an appointee is going to turn things around and implement a new agenda. From the bowels of the bureaucracy, however, can be heard the chorus of cynicism: "We were here when they arrived, and we'll be here when they leave."

It's not all their fault. Since about 1960, whenever anything goes wrong, the media pounces on a politician for an explanation or excuse that can be broadcast in 45 seconds or less. Usually, the politician states that they will introduce legislation to solve the problem, which can almost never be solved with legislation. The legislation, once enacted, almost always empowers a government agency to adopt regulations and take action.

Federal statutes and regulations have grown until they now total about 100 million words. The federal government estimates that people trying to comply with its purchasing procedures consume 289 million hours each year. The emphasis is on process rather than product. The bureaucrats who survive and thrive in this environment are the ones who keep their heads down, their voices quiet and their names out of the newspapers. After a few mind-numbing years of rolling with the tides, they stop wondering whether the time they spend on the job, or the job itself, has any impact on the mission of the agency they work for.

The administrative part of government thus has become a product of rat calculus. That is, the fourth branch of government has become a parody of itself, and the process of running through its self-created maze has become more important and interesting than asking whether the maze does any good.

What brings this to mind is the report of the Blue Ribbon Panel appointed by James Lee Witt, director of the Federal Emergency Management Agency (FEMA). The report, issued last October, is a wonderful document -probably the most lucid observations ever published about the 20-year deterioration of federal fire programs under FEMA's control. Steve Austin, representing the International Association of Arson Investigators, and Steve Edwards, director of the Maryland Fire and Rescue Institute, co-chaired the esteemed 13-member panel.

Consider the comments that appear on page 17 of the report: "The panel hopes that the leadership of FEMA can direct an organizational sea change in the agency in the recognition that fire/EMS provide the backbone of emergency preparedness and response in every community in America."

What a wonderful vision. I couldn't have said it better, but consider this: The leadership of FEMA is Witt. He's been more effective than his predecessors because he's got his head on straight; he's credible; he has basic leadership skills and a lot of energy; and he's close to the president.

FEMA is full of bureaucrats who have lots of experience in rat calculus. Many of them came to FEMA from other federal agencies. They're in the business of process. Instinctively, they dislike the way firefighters try to get things done (heads up, names in the newspaper and loud voices telling it like it is). Slowly, quietly undermining the U.S. Fire Administration and the National Fire Academy has become a part of the FEMA culture. Organizational cultures are deep-seated and tenacious. Witt is a short-timer; he cannot change the culture of FEMA before he leaves.

Any marriage between the fire service and the fourth branch of government is sure to produce ugly children. Maybe there's a better way.

Hoops, Loops and Mazes

In 1985, a lawsuit filed by a San Antonio city bus driver reached the U.S. Supreme Court. The court ruled that under the Fair Labor Standards Act (FLSA) public employees are entitled to time-and-a-half pay for overtime. The Court left the details of implementation to the bureaucracy-in this case, the U.S. Department of Labor (DOL). The DOL then developed regulations with the force and effect of law.

I knew we were in trouble when I attended a DOL workshop in 1986. A fire chief told the ranking DOL bureaucrat in attendance of a fire prevention inspector who routinely brought his lunch to the office and worked at his desk while eating.

"He cannot do that," warned the bureaucrat.

"I'm not making him work during his lunch hour," the chief replied. "He's just a dedicated guy, and he enjoys reading reports and doing paperwork while he eats lunch."

"Unless you want to pay him time-and-a-half for that hour," replied the bureaucrat, "you must instruct him in writing not to work while eating his lunch." So much for the work ethic, I thought as I listened to this exchange.

Somehow, most of us missed another bit of the DOL's fine

print-the 80/20 rule. This rule excludes from the Section 7(k) exemption those employees who spend less than 80 percent of their work time on activities related to fire and rescue. Their overtime pay would kick in at 40 hours rather than the 53-hour standard that applies to firefighters.

For public employees whose duties are limited to EMS, the 80/20 rule seems clear-cut. However, regarding cross-trained, multiple-role firefighter/paramedics, there has been confusion. Several lawsuits by public employees have proven two things: There is a price to be paid for every legal victory, and we cannot expect court rulings to clarify complex issues.

For nearly 30 years, the fire service has worked to broaden its responsibilities, mostly through cross training and multiple roles. In other words, we use firefighters for more than one public health and safety function. Thus, the marginal costs of a fire department EMS system using career employees usually are less than those of a private ambulance company. However, if those firefighters are entitled to overtime based on the 40-hour week, the economic advantage diminishes or disappears.

Commendably, the International Association of Fire Fighters (IAFF) has been out in front trying to resolve questions about the 80/20 rule. In February 1995, the administrator of the DOL's Employment Standards Administration wrote IAFF President Al Whitehead with an official clarification of the 80/20 rule.

According to the DOL letter, a cross-trained firefighter qualifies for the 7(k) exemption if "employed by an organized fire department or fire district ... trained to the extent required by state statute or ordinance ... has the legal authority and responsibility to engage in the prevention, control or extinguishment of a fire of any type. ... (This) term also includes rescue and ambulance personnel that form an integral part of the public agency's fire protection activities."

Here's the best part of the DOL letter: "Under these circumstances, we would consider that ambulance and rescue activities are incidental to the employees' fire protection duties ... (and) the time engaged in ambulance and rescue activities would be considered to be work performed as an incident to or in conjunction with the employees' fire protection activities ... and would not count in the 20-percent limitation on non-exempt work."

That should have settled it, but it didn't. So here's the picture. Congress (the legislative branch) enacted the FLSA in 1938. The Supreme Court (the judicial branch) interpreted a portion of the FLSA in 1985 and handed that interpretation over to the Department of Labor (the executive branch) for implementation. In 1986, the bureaucratic branch of the DOL adopted regulations that were in some respects arbitrary and confusing. Those regulations found their way back to the judicial branch after lawsuits were filed. In 1995, the executive branch (DOL) tried to clarify things with a letter, but its bureaucratic branch didn't bother to amend the DOL's own regulations. The confusion, the lawsuits and the inconsistent court rulings continued.

We've come full circle. By the time you read this, Maryland Congressman Robert Erlich will have introduced the FLSA Fire and Emergency Services Definition Act. Congressman Erlich deserves our gratitude and his legislation deserves our strong support.

At the same time, this whole episode is an example of why people are cynical about government. Somewhere in the DOL bureaucracy is a person who wrote the regulation that created this mess. Does that person ever talk to the high-level DOL bureaucrat who wrote the 1995 clarification letter? Why wasn't that letter followed by an effort to amend and clarify the regulations?

Recently, at an event sponsored by the Congressional Fire Services Institute, Congressman Curt Weldon advised attendees not to look for common sense in Washington. The 80/20 rule is a perfect example. Over the years, all three (or four) branches of government have managed to create, debate, articulate, interpret, confuse, arbitrate and obfuscate an issue that could have been resolved in about five minutes with common sense.

To the people who feed on your tax dollars and mine, the

process is more important than the outcome. The processes of each branch of government feed the processes of the others. The process of running through the hoops, loops and mazes has become more important than asking whether it does any good. It's rat calculus, and it's threatening the world's greatest experiment in representative government.

12

Movies and Television

Backdraft

Let's face it. Fires don't burn that way. A backdraft condition in a residential building doesn't shower the neighborhood with burning phosphorus. Although powerful, it doesn't pick someone up and thrust him headfirst through the windshield of a car parked in the street. A fire in a clothing factory does not confront firefighters with rogue fireballs that seem to travel from room to room in search of victims.

Even in the old days, firefighters couldn't work-much less breathe-in superheated building interiors for long periods without breathing apparatus, as flames licked at them from all sides. I don't know how it is in Chicago, but most off-duty firefighters would never get drunk and disorderly in their uniforms. And most firefighters would never start an auto extrication by running a saw diagonally through the driver's door.

But who cares? I spent my seven bucks to be entertained, and Ron Howard's film, "Backdraft," gave me my seven bucks' worth.

It's very difficult for me to get caught up in a movie. I'm always looking for technical details, flaws in the lighting or staging, editing mismatches and dubbed dialogue. Watching "Backdraft," it was only a minute until I was full absorbed in the story and the excitement. There may have been some technical flaws, but I didn't see them. What I did see was very powerful use of film and special effects, believable acting, an almost-believable story line, and a pace that held my attention.

Early in the film I thought Lt. Steve McCaffery's part was overplayed by actor Kurt Russell. But then I remembered a guy I had known who was very much like that. He was very unhappy, with a fragile ego and a chip on his shoulder. His whole identity was wrapped up in his reputation as a firefighter. He loved to make others the butt of his jokes but he couldn't take it in return. He took a lot of chances on the fire ground but, eventually, it was booze that killed him.

Actor William Baldwin played the role of probationary firefighter Brain McCaffery to a tee. It was a difficult role, requiring a full range of emotions, and he was believable in all of them except for some of the fire-combat heroics.

There was a retirement-party scene that must have been filmed at an actual retirement party. It had that feel to it. When a fistfight broke out, I first thought that it was a little far-fetched. Then I remembered a guy I used to work with. He couldn't handle his booze and, at fire department social functions, he would often get into fistfights. Eventually, they made him a chief and he stopped punching people.

One of the major plots in "Backdraft" dealt with a Chicago alderman's scheme to become mayor by reducing the cost of fire protection. He put together a phony team of consultants and they recommended closing some fire stations. We watched as the big fires got bigger, and no backup fire companies were available (due to the cutbacks).

Eventually, the fire investigator, played by Robert De Niro, stormed into a press conference being held by the crooked alderman. He disclosed the evidence that the alderman's consultants were actually his secret business associates, and the man's mayoral campaign came to an abrupt end.

I loved the scene in "Backdraft" in which a Mercedes was

parked in front of a hydrant. Engine 17's crew ran a suction hose in the driver's window and out the passenger's window to make their hookup. Who among us has not yearned for such an opportunity?

Old engine drivers are a breed apart and there has never been an actor who could properly imitate one. Engine 17's driver in "Backdraft" added a lot of realism-fat and grouchy, crusty as a barnacle, with a croak for a voice. He must have been one of the Chicago firefighters who was pressed into service as an actor.

In the background of one fire-station scene, a sign on the wall said: "Chicago Fire Department: 150 Years of Tradition Unimpeded by Progress." The film reinforced CFD's reputation as a traditional blue-collar organization. Like it or not, setting the film in the Chicago Fire Department gave the film a lot of texture that couldn't be found elsewhere.

Lots of our colleagues will criticize lots of technical details in "Backdraft," including the gross violation of every known safety standard. However, they need to realize that actors can't be filmed through real smoke, that audiences wouldn't tolerate two hours of dialogue though the face pieces of breathing apparatus, and that there's a big difference between training and entertainment. This is not a training film.

I'll limit my criticism to the prevalence of cigarette smoking by the firefighters in the film. It wasn't essential to the story. If the people at CFD who advised Ron Howard had had any interest in firefighter health and safety, they would have discouraged it. The scenes of firefighters lighting up while overhauling a fire, or an engine driver behind the wheel with a cigarette dangling from his mouth, bother those of us who've seen too many firefighters die prematurely from the effects of smoking.

If you haven't already seen it, and if you're looking for some entertainment (rather than training or education), I would encourage you to rent the video "Backdraft."

Real Life Became Drama

About the time the TV show "Rescue 911" announced it would continue broadcasting for another season, the Los Angeles Times published a story that brought back a flood of memories. It was about a little girl named Kathy Fiscus.

Long before Andy Warhol observed that each of us is likely to have 15 minutes of fame, a handful of rescuers achieved fame unlike anything previously seen. On a weekend four decades before "Rescue 911" came along, most of the 20,000 TV sets in the Los Angeles area were tuned day and night to riveting drama of an intensely difficult effort to save a life.

It was April 9, 1949. My Dad had recently purchased our first TV set, and I was among those who couldn't resist watching the 27-hour continuous broadcast. It all started on a Friday evening. Three-year-old Kathy Fiscus had been running through the tall green grass of a vacant lot in the LA suburb of San Marino. In an instant, the child disappeared into the open shaft of an abandoned well.

When Alice Fiscus began searching for her daughter, she heard faint cries from the well. She called the local fire department. The well casing was 100 feet deep and only 14 inches in diameter. Firefighters set up a hand-powered air pump and slipped an air hose and the end of a rope down the shaft. Kathy grabbed the rope and was pulled up a few feet, but she lost her grip and slid to a spot 94 feet below the ground.

It was decided that a parallel shaft was needed and the digging began. About that time, the manager of KTLA, one of the area's first television stations, decided to send sportscaster Bill Welsh and special events announcer Stan Chambers to the scene. The Kathy Fiscus rescue effort was to become television's first live coverage of a news event.

A friend called us on the phone. "Do you have a TV?" She asked. We were already watching the rescue effort on the tiny black-and -white screen, frequently adjusting the vertical hold knob to keep the picture from tumbling. Despite the hazy images on the primitive TV set, we were tense as we watched the rescue effort grow. The tension mounted when Welsh announced with a quaking voice that the sides of the parallel shaft had crumbled as workers tried to descent into it.

Another shaft was started, however, and our hopes were raised. Stan Chambers held up a photograph of grinning Kathy Fiscus in a pretty white dress. The camera moved in close on the photo. She was no longer a stranger; Kathy Fiscus became the first visual image of a life-threatened person to be electronically transmitted to our living room. Instantly, we felt a bond with the child and her parents.

Then came word that the second parallel shaft was filling with water. Forty-five years later, I can remember the hollow feeling of disappointment. Then Bill Welsh broadcast a call for volunteers to help. Again, our hopes were restored. Surely, we thought, among all the people watching this extraordinary event, there would be someone with some kind of magic solution.

Before it was over, 132 volunteers came forth. They included a former coal miner, a former Navy diver, several jockeys willing to be lowered into the shaft, and an unemployed construction foreman named Yancey. The broadcasters gave several of these people their few minutes of fame. More than the others, though, they made Yancey a celebrity of sorts, especially after it was learned that he borrowed streetcar fare to get to the scene.

Fifty hours after Mrs. Fiscus' first call for help, rescuers completed the parallel shaft and cut through the pipe. I'll never forget the suspense as we waited for a report on Kathy's condition. We held our breath...as though it might a difference. Then came the news that Kathy was dead. I was 13 and self-conscious; I left the room before my family could see me cry.

The years since 1949 have seen improvements in rescue training, equipment and incident command. We all remember a similar incident several years ago in Waco, Texas. Fortunately, Jessica McClure survived her ordeal in an unprotected well casing, and the story of her rescue became a TV movie.

There's a bronze marker behind San Marino's city library in memory of Kathy Fiscus. It refers to "a little girl who brought the world together-for a moment." Indeed, when we stop to think of the subsequent impact of live, on-the-scene news reporting it seems that one little girl's death triggered enormous changes in the way we view the world.

The American public remains fascinated with rescues and rescuers. But the TV cameras and those who report and edit the stories have acquired a hard, cynical edge in the years since the rescue of Kathy Fiscus.

In 1949, real life became drama portrayed through a TV screen. Today, drama creates images that people confuse with real life. All the more reason for every rescuer to be trained, equipped and organized for the worst of situations.

Greed for a Good Cause

One of my favorite hobbies is working with the County of Los Angeles Fire Museum Association. Presently, we have 32 antique fire apparatus (including the newly restored Squad 51 from "Emergency!") and lots of artifacts that document the history of the fire service generally and the Los Angeles County Fire Department specifically. The Association stores most of these items in an old warehouse in a tough part of town.

The Museum Association board of directors meets monthly in the dusty, unheated warehouse. Our primary meeting topic is finding and funding a permanent home for the collection. Unfortunately, the down payment on the kind of facility we want would equal about $1 million, which, of course, the Association doesn't have.

This past November, I mentioned to my wife that I needed to find a million or more dollars for the Association. A few days later, she directed my attention to a *Los Angeles Times* ad. The television game show "Greed" wanted contestants.

"I couldn't do that," I protested. "Imagine what would happen to my reputation if I appeared on a game show called 'Greed'.

"Well, you said you needed a million dollars," she replied,

"and your grandsons think you're the smartest person in the world." (Occasionally, the boys and I watch "Jeopardy" together, and sometimes I come up with correct responses.)

I thought about it for several days. Then, in an impulsive moment, I called the phone number in the ad. An answering machine picked up. I left my name and phone number, but I really didn't expect to hear from them.

About a week later, I got a phone call from a pleasant young woman named Melissa. She wanted to give me an appointment for an audition. We settled on 6 p.m., Dec. 15. I hung up the phone and thought, 'Uh oh, this is getting out of control'."

Days before the audition, I fretted a lot. I imagined friends, enemies and grandchildren watching their TVs as I engaged in greedy competition for something as tawdry and undignified as money. What if I missed an easy question and came home with my reputation tarnished and my pockets empty? But it's for a worthy cause, I argued (with myself).

On the 15th, during the three-hour drive to Hollywood, I nearly turned around at least a dozen times. To keep myself going, I envisioned a beautiful museum with polished floors, a research library and perfectly restored antique fire apparatus that visitors admired. Finally, I arrived at the TV studio about 5:30 p.m.

Already about 30 people had lined up on the sidewalk next to the studio gate. I went to the back of the line and struck up a conversation with the people around me. I was pleasantly surprised to find normal working folks who shared some of my apprehensions and embarrassment. By 6 p.m., about 50 of us had congregated, and a guy with a clipboard worked his way down the line, checking off names.

At 6:15, they ushered us in the gate and asked us to gather around a young guy with long hair who stood on a box in a paved area between sound stages (barn-like structures where they film TV shows). He gave us a short explanation of what would happen, and then he randomly put us into groups of six. Two young women, including Melissa, then led each group into a sound stage. The sound stage was painted black on the inside, and the temperature was about 60 degrees. We saw several rows of picnic tables with seats. A studio crew member guided each group of six to its respective bench and seated it.

Applications and test answer sheets were on the tables in front of each person. They told us we would receive a 24-question multiple-choice test. One of the young women would ask a question, then state the possible answers. Without hesitation, she would ask the question and state the possible answers a second time. If you didn't comprehend the question and enter the correct answer by the time she went to the next question, it was too bad.

Immediately after she had asked the last question, our tester told us to leave our answer sheets on the bench, and, under escort, all 50 of us went outdoors to the open area. Within 10 minutes, Melissa and her partner came out with the list of those who had passed the test. One by one, they called 12 names, including mine. Unceremoniously, the other 38 people left.

The 12 of us went back to the sound stage and took our seats at the tables where we had taken the test. In front of the tables sat a mock-up of the "Greed" stage: four lecterns and a place for the captain to stand. We also saw a small stand with two buttons on it for the *Terminator* contests.

There's more to the story, and if you've ever dreamed of competing on a TV game show, you may find it interesting. I'll wrap it up in the next essay.

That's Show Biz

In the previous essay, I shared the story of my audition for a television game show called "Greed." My goal was to win a million bucks for the County of Los Angeles Fire Museum Association. The museum, which houses several rigs that I worked on during my career as a firefighter, needs a permanent home.

The museum and its needs are a frequent topic of conversation at our house. So, when my wife spotted an ad last November for game-show contestants, she suggested I apply. Reluctantly, I began the process and on December 15 drove to Hollywood for a test and audition. Fifty people took the test, and 12 of us survived.

For a few moments, I felt sorry for the 38 people who failed the test. They walked out the gate stunned and silent. As a firefighter, television advisor and writer, I've worked in and around Hollywood and I know how brutal the town can be. On the other hand, their departure meant only 12 of us remained to compete for the million bucks. That's what I was thinking as we walked into a mock-up of the "Greed" stage.

A pleasant middle-age woman introduced herself as the contestant coordinator. She said she'd done that job for many years and had worked on some of the best-known game shows in

Hollywood. She was looking for good projection, poise under pressure, personality, etc. Glancing at the other contestants, I thought, "I'm in!"

The pleasant lady then led us through several mock games of "Greed." Luckily, I wasn't in the first group, which gave me a chance to learn from the others' mistakes. Raphael, a Cuban-American with a soft voice and a thick Spanish accent, was the first group's captain. When asked to speak up, Raphael was difficult to hear or understand. I couldn't imagine he'd be selected for the show.

Also in the first group was Chris, our "valedictorian," who got the highest score on the test. He had a shaved head and wore a big earring. When asked to identify and describe himself for the group, he said he was in the liquor-distribution business. Three times during the interview process, he admitted to being a functioning alcoholic. I wasn't sure whether he was kidding, but I figured it would eliminate him from the competition.

I was chosen for the second presentation and was appointed captain. I identified myself simply as a retired firefighter. My team included another tall, bald, middle-age guy-a car salesman named Bruce. As our mock game began, members of the "Greed" staff watched and took notes. The first few questions were easy. Then the Terminator round landed on the car salesman, who then challenged me.

It was quite a scene. Two competitive, Type-A guys, right hands poised over the kill buttons, waiting for the question. "Who was the first U.S. President to be born in the 20th century?" Somehow, from somewhere, the answer came to me before the coordinator finished reading the question: John F. Kennedy. I hit the button and the car salesman's jaw dropped.

The remaining three team members and I made it to the half-million-dollar level. Then came the question, "According to the Gallup Poll, which four of the following six presidents had approval ratings of 80 percent or better? Bush, Clinton, FDR, JFK, Truman or Reagan?" As the captain, I changed my teammates' answer, and I was wrong. The correct answer was Bush, FDR, JFK and Truman.

Actually, none of the teams got past the $500,000-mark in practice. But the "Greed" staff assured us they weren't interested in how much make-believe money we made. They were sizing us up as performers. As the evening progressed, I assumed that only three or four from our group were contenders. One 24-year-old college student blurted out that he's a compulsive gambler who needs to win on "Greed" because all his credit cards are maxed out.

In the end, "Greed" coordinators told us we might hear from them sometime between Christmas and New Year's Day. They also said they have hundreds of eligible contestants and the Fox Network had purchased only seven additional one-hour broadcasts.

When I wrote the first part of this story, I really expected to get the call from "Greed" before writing the second installment. The call hasn't come yet. In January, I tuned into the TV show and saw Bruce the car salesman and Chris the functioning alcoholic. Both went home penniless. Go figure.

No matter what happens, it was a fascinating adventure. Meanwhile, some beautiful pieces of fire service history sit in a cold, dusty warehouse waiting for a permanent home. Maybe I should call Regis Philbin.

Epilogue

I Remember

I remember visiting with Ray Downey and his lovely wife in Sacramento earlier this year. FDNY's renowned rescue chief spoke at FDIC West, and he and his wife had taken some extra time to tour the Napa Valley wine country. They were relaxed and enjoying life and each other. Ray talked with pride about his two sons on the job. I'll never forget the hollow feeling when I heard ABC TV announce that Ray had been killed at the World Trade Center.

I remember taking my sister on a tour of the World Trade Center years ago. We marveled at the long elevator ride and then the spectacular view from the top.

I remember a dinner at the Windows on the World restaurant in the 1980s. I don't remember much about the meal. It was eclipsed by the whole experience of sitting next to a window a quarter-mile above the street.

I remember writing about a trip into New York 19 years ago.[1] I got on the wrong subway train and ended up beneath the World Trade Center rather than my intended stop. After squeezing into the herd that inched its way to the escalators leading to the street, I wondered how people could endure those rigors every workday—year after year—and retain their sanity.

I remember the rationing of gasoline, tires, sugar, butter and meat during World War II, and I remember my family enduring deprivation with a sense of patriotic pride. I wonder if the current generation of Americans is willing to endure such inconveniences for more than a month or two.

I remember my mother crying when the Korean War started. She and her generation had already lived through two world wars. Her son was three years shy of draft age. I wonder how many mothers cried on Sept. 11, 2001.

I remember trying to explain to my young sons how and why our next-door neighbors' son was killed during the Tet Offensive in a far-off place called Vietnam. I remember thinking that war is never so ugly as when you try to explain it to a child.

I remember commercial aviation before security screening existed. I remember getting to airports with a few minutes to spare and always catching my flight. Never again will that be possible.

I remember standing in airport boarding lounges and paying no attention to the other people who would fly with me. I detest prejudice, but how can I not be suspicious of fellow passengers who speak in foreign tongues or who look like those recently identified as terrorists?

I remember going through airport security checkpoints and watching minimum-wage personnel visiting with each other, paying no attention to the monitor that would reveal the contents of my carry-on bag. If it happens again, should I report them to someone or mind my own business? If my own safety while flying is not my business, whose is it?

I remember publishing an editorial about terrorism nearly 20 years ago. It was ahead of its time, and readers told us so; but one paragraph in particular seems worth repeating:

> *"The ultimate goal of terrorists is to destroy the fabric of free societies. In North America, that fabric is fortified by the resolve of people to care for and about one another. Modern*

emergency services are some of the best weapons against the ultimate goals of those who would destroy our social structure. It is all about caring and doing for others what we would want done for ourselves in similar circumstances."[2]

I remember an article in the Wall Street Journal (WSJ) last February. It portrayed firefighters as too numerous and without enough legitimate work. If you've never been to New York, you may not know that Wall Street is a few hundred feet from where the World Trade Center stood. It would seem appropriate for the WSJ to now honor those firefighters who lost their lives running into buildings that others were running out of.

[1] *"Stress and Strain," The Publisher's Page, JEMS, October 1982*

[2] *"The Threat of Terrorism," Editorial, JEMS, February 1982*

Separating the Men from the Boys

Would you have sent people into those buildings?" my wife asked as we watched another replay of the Twin Towers burning. "You're damn right I would," I snapped. "Would you have gone in those buildings yourself?" she asked. "Of course—that's what the job is all about," I replied. "I'm glad I didn't know you then," she added softly.

A few days later I received a note from Paul Carmichael, a retired firefighter I worked with at Station 7 in West Hollywood. He sent along an old photo of us in front of the station. Paul had played for the Denver Broncos before joining our fire department. He was strong, smart and totally reliable. "We were a good crew," Paul's note said.

In the fire service, we always like to think we're part of a good crew. But you never really know until you face the kind of test that distinguishes firefighters from regular people. Paul and I faced that kind of test one night. We were first-in on one of the West Coast's first high-rise fires—and the nearest chief officer was nearly 30 minutes away.

Though only 10 stories tall, the building's third through sixth floors were fully involved when we arrived. As I climbed off the engine, the building's night watchman told me people on the top floor were trapped and screaming for help. As incident commander, I ordered Paul and two other firefighters to conduct a search-and-rescue operation.

At a moment like that, a man's eyes tell a lot. To this day, I can remember looking into those guys' faces as they donned their breathing apparatus. Regular people would have shown some sign of apprehension. After all, the building was burning and they would have to make their way through the fire to reach the victims. But those guys were not regular people. Their eyes showed gritty determination to save the lives of some complete strangers.

They made it to the top floor only to find the night watchman had been hallucinating. There were no victims to rescue. But my crew hadn't known that when they ran into that burning high-rise. In less than a minute, they had arrived at the biggest fire they'd ever seen, received an order that was inherently dangerous and followed that order without question or hesitation.

A few days after receiving Paul's note, I got a call from a well-known fire chief. He asked me what I was hearing about firefighters being fearful or apprehensive in the aftermath of Sept. 11. I said I hadn't heard anything of that nature, but I had been wondering about those people who joined the fire service primarily for the work schedule, the benefits and the pension system. Could they be counted on when things got really dangerous?

Then I read the transcript of testimony recently given by a firefighter in a hearing. His department's EMS coordinator had failed to renew the firefighter's automated external defibrillator (AED) certification in a timely manner. The firefighter testified he wouldn't use the defibrillator unless his certification was current because he feared being sued and didn't believe his department would back him.

In other words, at least one American firefighter would allow a pulseless, non breathing patient to slip away because he fears a lawsuit. Never mind that AEDs hang on the walls of airports, malls, stadiums and any number of public places, available for ordinary citizens to use. Never mind that a pulseless, non-breathing person is already clinically dead; thus, there's no basis for a lawsuit if they remain dead. Never mind that every state has immunity ("Good Samaritan") laws to protect good faith rescuers from liability.

As I read that testimony, I thought of the 343 firefighters who ran into the Twin Towers and died there. I'm sure they had that same look of determination I saw on the face of Paul Carmichael and our colleagues that night on Sunset Boulevard. I'm sure they would have answered my wife's question as I did. I'm sure they would feel as I do about reluctant rescuers.

There's not much good to find in the events of Sept. 11. But it may have forced us to take stock of firefighting and rescue after three decades of political correctness and social engineering.

If you call yourself a firefighter and you're not willing to risk your life to save a stranger, turn in your badge. If you joined a fire department primarily for the salary, security, convenience, social life or any other selfish motive, step aside and make room for a real firefighter. If you would hesitate to rescue a dying person because you're afraid of a lawsuit, go get a job as a social worker or an accountant—you're in the wrong business.

More than 4,800 American firefighters have died in the line of duty since I first earned the right to call myself a firefighter. The public respect and adoration we now enjoy was paid for with those priceless lives. Nobody has a right to bask in that respect and adoration unless they're willing to confront all manner of risks in the service of others—without hesitation, qualification or negotiation. Anything less insults the memory of those who have made the ultimate sacrifice.